The South Beach Diet

Of 2024

The Ultimate Guide to Effortless and Healthy Weight Loss for Improved Health

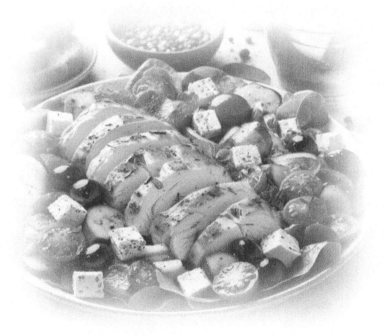

Kristy Nolan

TABLE OF CONTENTS

Book Introduction

Here is a thorough handbook that will change the way you think about health and weight loss: "The South Beach Diet of 2024: A Faster, Easier, and Delicious Plan for Improved Health and Weight Loss." In these pages, you'll find a refined and evolved diet, suited to the demands of contemporary lifestyles, that is widely recognized for its effectiveness and flexibility.

Accepting a Healthy You

The South Beach Diet has a long history of changing people's lives because it provides a balanced approach that puts long-term lifestyle changes ahead of fads. This updated version, which incorporates the most recent research and nutritional expertise, upholds the fundamental concepts of the original while also incorporating breakthroughs and insights. The year is 2024.

Adapting for the Best Outcomes

The South Beach Diet has evolved thoughtfully in its current form to meet the ever-changing demands and obstacles experienced by those attempting to maintain long-term weight loss and better health. The 2024 version offers a more simplified, effective, and pleasurable route to success by carefully taking into account scientific advancements, dietary trends, and real-world input.

What Is Unique About 2024

Unlike its predecessors, the 2024 edition offers a number of crucial improvements:

Precision in Nutrition: A greater comprehension of nutritional science has improved the structure of the diet and ensured a more accurate distribution of vital macronutrients.

Personalized Approach: This revised edition welcomes personalization, acknowledging that each person is unique and providing flexible tactics to suit a range of dietary needs and lifestyles.

Enhanced Flexibility: The foundation of the updated South Beach Diet is flexibility. It preserves its core ideas while enabling a smoother integration into hectic schedules.

Objectives and Advantages

The empowerment of people to attain optimal health and long-term weight management is still the core objective of the South Beach Diet. By following its tenets, participants stand to gain a variety of advantages:

Effective Weight Loss: Reduce extra weight in a consistent, healthful manner without sacrificing vital nutrients or feeling starved.

Better Metabolic Health: The diet's concentration on a balanced food helps to improve metabolic health by regulating blood sugar and boosting energy levels.

Enhanced Well-Being: In addition to losing weight, people say they feel more invigorated, have better mental clarity, and have a general sense of wellbeing.

The Road Ahead

This article will provide you with a thorough grasp of the South Beach Diet in its 2024 iteration before you set off on this life-changing journey. We explore the ins and outs of the diet's processes, meal plans, and success tactics in a number of coherent chapters.

A Guarantee of Outcomes

The success stories that are presented in these pages attest to the South Beach Diet's efficacy. These real-life makeovers inspire and motivate by showing that maintaining good health and controlling weight are achievable objectives.

Accepting Change for a Better Future

In summary, rather than just being a diet plan, "The South Beach Diet of 2024" is a lifestyle shift that prioritizes your long-term health. Accepting change and putting this guide's lessons into practice can help you go in the right direction and live a better, happier life today.

Come along as we examine the subtleties, advantages, and real-world applications of this modified South Beach Diet, helping you to control your weight sustainably and achieve better health in the ever-changing year 2024 and beyond.

CHAPTER 1
Overview of the 2024 South Beach Diet

Introducing the updated and rejuvenated South Beach Diet, a modern interpretation of the well-known eating strategy designed for optimum health and weight control in 2024. We take you on a fascinating journey through the guiding ideas, development, and essential concepts that characterize the most recent version of the South Beach Diet in this chapter, equipping you with the knowledge you need to make a life-changing decision.

The Origins of the South Beach Diet: A Famous doctor developed the South Beach Diet, which rose to popularity in the early 2000s due to its well-balanced approach to nutrition that prioritizes food quality over rigorous calorie tracking. It was created in response to the demand for a long-term, health-oriented diet that prioritized general wellbeing over short-term weight loss.

The Foundation of the South Beach Diet: The South Beach Diet is based on the idea of substituting better options for "bad" fats and "bad" carbohydrates. It promotes consuming whole grains, lean proteins, and foods high in fiber in moderation and limiting processed carbs and harmful fats. Blood sugar levels should be stabilized, cravings should be lessened, and a sustainable, balanced eating pattern should be encouraged.

Development in 2024: The South Beach Diet has experienced a deliberate development in 2024. With a focus on human physiology, behavioral psychology, and nutritional science, this version provides a more sophisticated and flexible method to meet the changing demands of those looking for long-term weight management and better health.

What's Novel:

The South Beach Diet undergoes numerous significant improvements in 2024.

Precision in Nutrition: New scientific understandings have refined the macronutrient composition of the diet while highlighting the significance of consuming a high-quality, nutrient-dense diet.

Personalized Approach: The revised South Beach Diet provides a more flexible framework that takes into account people's particular tastes, nutritional needs, and lifestyles. It does this by acknowledging that every person is unique.

Flexibility and Accessibility: The 2024 edition has a strong emphasis on flexibility in order to better accommodate a variety of schedules without compromising the diet's core principles. This is in recognition of the demands of modern living.

The South Beach Diet's Scientific Basis

The scientific basis of the South Beach Diet is essential to its effectiveness. Through insulin regulation and blood sugar stabilization, the diet encourages fat loss without compromising muscle mass. The focus on nutrient-dense foods also promotes heart health, brain function, and increased energy levels, among other aspects of general wellness.

It's critical to approach the South Beach Diet with reasonable expectations. Set realistic expectations. Although many people want to lose weight, the diet prioritizes long-term lifestyle adjustments above temporary cures. It is anticipated that participants will make consistent, incremental progress toward their health goals.

As we come to the end of this first chapter, it should be clear that the South Beach Diet of 2024 is a sophisticated, scientifically supported strategy for promoting long-term weight management and overall health rather than a fad. Further exploration of the mechanisms, phases, meal plans, and tactics for success within this modified dietary framework will take place in the upcoming chapters.

CHAPTER 2
The South Beach Diet's Development: What's New in 2024

This chapter delves into the evolution of the South Beach Diet, examining the revolutionary additions and changes that characterize the 2024 iteration. The South Beach Diet has been painstakingly modified to meet the requirements and goals of people who are currently pursuing better health and long-term weight control, building on its rich history and strong basis.

Changing with the Times: The South Beach Diet has always accepted change, modifying itself to take into account new dietary understandings, scientific advancements, and shifting lifestyle patterns. This versatility distinguishes 2024 from its predecessors in a number of revolutionary ways.

Accuracy in Nutrition: A notable development of the South Beach Diet is its increased accuracy in nutritional advice. The importance of maintaining an ideal macronutrient balance is emphasized in the 2024 version. It emphasizes the importance of lipids, proteins, and carbs once again and promotes complete, unprocessed meals high in nutrients with low levels of harmful fats and refined carbohydrates.

Personalization and Flexibility: The 2024 edition has a more customized strategy than earlier iterations. Since each person has different dietary requirements and interests, the diet provides a range of customized possibilities. It allows individuals to customize the diet to fit their specific needs while adhering to its fundamental principles. It also takes into account a variety of nutritional requirements, cultural preferences, and lifestyles.

Technological Integration: The South Beach Diet of 2024 makes use of technology to improve user experience in an era dominated by technological developments. The program incorporates mobile applications, interactive tools, and user-friendly interfaces to make monitoring simpler, offer individualized recommendations, and connect users with a community of support, all of which promote responsibility and incentive.

Accepting Behavioral Science: The 2024 edition integrates behavioral science concepts because it recognizes that effective dietary modifications involve more than just food selections. It provides methods for overcoming psychological obstacles, routines, and emotional eating tendencies. Participants are better prepared to execute and sustain dietary changes in a sustainable manner by cultivating a positive mentality and rewarding healthy habits.

Sustainability and Longevity: The South Beach Diet of 2024 promotes sustainable eating choices in keeping with the growing emphasis on sustainable living. It highlights the use of seasonally appropriate, locally grown produce and raises awareness of environmental effect. The diet supports sustainable eating practices and mindfulness, which are in line with both individual health objectives and larger environmental concerns.

Integration of State-of-the-Art Research: The South Beach Diet's 2024 progression is supported by state-of-the-art research and is not coincidental. The new guidelines are based on a comprehensive review of nutritional studies, clinical trials, and behavioral research, ensuring that recommendations are supported by scientific evidence.

With its 2024 version, the South Beach Diet is more than simply a diet plan; it's a holistic approach to health that takes into account advances in technology, nutrition, behavioral science, and sustainability. This evolution, which is based on adaptability and research, is to empower people on their path to better health and long-term weight management.

CHAPTER 3
The Workings of the South Beach Diet

Comprehending the concepts and mechanisms that facilitate the South Beach Diet's operation is crucial for its effective execution and compliance. This chapter tries to clarify the basic principles and procedures of the diet, providing information that will help you maintain your weight loss and enhance your health.

The Trilogy of Stages

The three main phases of the South Beach Diet, each intended to fulfill a specific purpose in reaching nutritional and health goals, constitute the foundation of the program:

Phase One: Reset Your Body: This two-week period is dedicated to getting rid of cravings and bringing your blood sugar levels back to normal. Participants consume lean meats, healthy fats, and vegetables high in fiber while dramatically reducing their diet of carbohydrates, sweets, and starches with a high glycemic index.

Phase Two: Reintroducing Carbs and Maintaining Weight Loss: In this phase, whole grains, fruits, and some starchy vegetables are prioritized as a way to gradually reintroduce nutritious carbohydrates into the diet. This stage lasts until the person achieves their target weight.

Phase Three: Maintenance and Healthy Lifestyle: Maintaining the dietary guidelines acquired over the preceding two phases is what defines this last stage. It places a strong emphasis on maintaining long-term weight loss and general wellbeing through consistent exercise, portion control, and nutritious food.

Macronutrient Balancing: The South Beach Diet limits the intake of macronutrients while emphasizing the consumption of nutrient-dense foods.

Healthy Fats: Including healthy fats in the diet, such as those in nuts, seeds, avocados, and olive oil, is essential for promoting general health, satiety, and nutrient absorption.

Lean Proteins: Vital for maintaining muscle mass, metabolism, and satiety, meals high in proteins, like fish, chicken, lentils, and tofu, are included in each phase.

Good Carbohydrates: Reintroducing whole grains, fruits, and some vegetables as well as other good carbs at later stages can provide a balanced intake of nutrients that provide energy without quickly raising blood sugar levels.

Control of Insulin and Blood Sugar: The South Beach Diet's influence on insulin levels is a fundamental component. To balance insulin levels, the diet restricts high-glycemic-index carbs during Phase One and then progressively adds them back later. This regulation aids in lowering cravings, regulating appetite, and encouraging fat burning.

The diet places a strong emphasis on consuming entire, unprocessed foods rather than their refined alternatives. Whole foods increase metabolism, aid in better digestion, and are high in antioxidants, fiber, and other minerals. They also promote general health.

Prolonged Health and Welfare

The South Beach Diet places a high priority on general health and wellbeing in addition to weight loss. Its focus on nutrient-dense meals, a balanced intake of macronutrients, and sustainable lifestyle modifications are in line with more general health goals including better blood sugar regulation, heart health, and enhanced energy.

Knowing the inner workings of the South Beach Diet emphasizes how well it works to support long-term, healthy weight maintenance. Its success is largely due to its scheduled phases, emphasis on nutrient-dense foods, and control over insulin levels. Following its guidelines can help people lose weight, improve their general well-being, and develop a healthy relationship with food.

CHAPTER 4
An Explanation of the Three Stages

The three phases of the South Beach Diet, which is well-known for its methodical approach, are specifically designed to aid in weight loss, stabilize blood sugar, and encourage long-term health. This chapter explores the specifics of each stage, explaining the goals, protocols, and food plans for each.

Phase One: Reset Your Body Objective

By regulating blood sugar levels and removing cravings for refined carbohydrates and sweets, Phase One aims to both jumpstart weight reduction and reset the body's response to food.

Rules:
When the first two weeks started:

Lean proteins, foods with a high fiber content, healthy fats, and low-glycemic index are the main emphasis of the participants.
Restrictions apply to fruits, starchy vegetables, processed carbs, and refined sugars.

Consuming three well-balanced meals and snacks on a regular basis can provide blood sugar stability and fullness.

Meal Organization:

Breakfast: Meals high in protein, such as eggs, Greek yogurt, or tofu, served with veggies and healthy fats.

Lunch consists of leafy greens, cruciferous vegetables, lean meats (fish or poultry), and a healthy fat source.

Dinner is akin to lunch, but with different options for vegetables and protein sources.

Snacks: To stave off hunger between meals, try hummus-topped veggie sticks, nuts, or seeds.

Results: Due to decreased insulin levels and decreased water retention, participants frequently report quick initial weight loss during this phase. Blood sugar levels that are stable also lead to less cravings and more energy.

Phase Two: Continued Weight Loss and the Reintroduction of Carbs

Goal: By progressively reintroducing healthful carbohydrates, Phase Two aims to expand dietary options and promote a long-term weight loss strategy.

Guidelines: Adhere to the Phase One guidelines and gradually introduce fruits, whole grains, and some starchy vegetables.

Keep an eye on each person's tolerance for carbs and modify consumption as necessary.

Maintain your mindful eating practices and portion management.

Meal Organization:

Breakfast: Include fruits, full grain cereals, or oatmeal with lean meats and healthy fats.

Lunch and dinner should consist of a variety of lean proteins and vegetables paired with nutritious grains, legumes, fruits, and starchy vegetables.

Snacks: To add variety to your snack selections, try adding fruits, whole grain crackers, or yogurt.

Results: During this phase, participants usually lose weight more slowly but steadily and have access to a wider variety of satisfying foods. Increased meal pleasure and heightened energy levels are factors that support the sustainability of the diet.

Phase Three: Sustaining and Leading a Healthful Lifestyle

Phase Three's goal is to help participants maintain their weight loss and develop a lifelong commitment to healthy eating by building on the habits they developed in the previous phases.

Guidelines: Prioritize portion control, regular physical activity, and eating balanced meals.

promotes consuming complete, nutrient-dense foods in excess occasionally but allows moderation for occasional indulgences.

encourages attentive eating practices and an understanding of bodily cues.

Meal Structure: Similar to Phase Two, but with some extra leeway and in moderation, on occasion.

To keep things interesting and avoid boredom, try out different dishes, cuisines, and culinary pairings.

Results: The goal of Phase Three is to develop a sustainable lifestyle that embraces a flexible and balanced approach to eating while guaranteeing weight maintenance. Individuals frequently report long-lasting weight loss, enhanced general health indicators, and an increased sense of control over their food choices.

The South Beach Diet's three phases provide a methodical but flexible way to lose weight and maintain a healthy lifestyle. People who follow these stages with dedication and comprehension not only reach their weight objectives but also have a better comprehension of long-term health tactics and balanced eating.

CHAPTER 5
The South Beach Diet's Advantages in 2024

In 2024, the South Beach Diet is still regarded as a thorough and successful eating strategy that goes much beyond weight loss. The numerous advantages that followers of this improved and modified diet can look forward to are discussed in this chapter.

Sustainable Weight Loss:

One of the South Beach Diet's most well-known features is how well it works to encourage long-term weight loss. With a focus on nutrient-dense foods, blood sugar stabilization, and smart insulin control, participants frequently see consistent, long-lasting weight loss without sacrificing vital nutrients or feeling deprived.

Better Metabolic Health:

The diet's beneficial effects on metabolic health are essential to its effectiveness. The South Beach Diet helps to improve metabolic indicators by controlling the insulin response and promoting the consumption of lean proteins, healthy fats, and complex carbs. Thus, improved metabolic health as a whole leads to improved blood sugar regulation and higher levels of energy.

Decreased appetites and Increased Satiety:

Participants frequently report a marked decrease in their appetites for processed and sugary meals during Phase One. Eating meals high in protein and healthy fats increases satiety, which lowers the risk of giving in to bad food urges. This decreased reliance on items with a high glycemic index aids in maintaining dietary modifications over time.

Heart Health and Blood Pressure Control:

Promoting heart-healthy fats, such as those in avocados, nuts, seeds, and olive oil, helps lower blood pressure. The diet lowers the risk of cardiovascular illnesses by encouraging the consumption of monounsaturated and polyunsaturated fats while restricting the intake of saturated and trans fats. This helps to control cholesterol levels.

Enhanced Energy and Mental Clarity:

As South Beach Diet participants move through the phases, many report feeling more energised and having better mental clarity. Blood sugar stabilization and nutrient-dense food consumption power the body and brain, providing long-lasting energy and improved cognitive performance.

Improved Digestive Wellness and Health:

Including fruits, vegetables, and whole grains high in fiber promotes digestive health by promoting regular bowel movements and preserving a healthy gut microbiota. This leads to better general health, which includes stronger immunity, decreased inflammation, and increased mood.

Sustainable Lifestyle Changes:

The South Beach Diet's capacity to promote sustainable lifestyle changes is arguably one of its most important advantages. Participants are given the tools to maintain long-term health and weight management by the diet, which teaches them about mindful eating, balanced nutrition, and the value of regular physical activity.

Beyond only helping people lose weight, the South Beach Diet of 2024 has many other advantages like greater heart health, decreased cravings, more energy, and long-lasting lifestyle adjustments. People who follow the guidelines of this diet can see a complete change in their entire health and well-being as well as in how they physically look.

CHAPTER 6
The South Beach Diet's Scientific Basis

Scientific principles and nutritional insights provide a strong foundation for the efficacy of the South Beach Diet. The scientific basis for the diet's workings is explained in this chapter, along with how it affects metabolism, controls insulin response, and promotes long-term weight loss.

Insulin Level Regulation: The South Beach Diet's primary focus is on insulin regulation, which is essential for blood sugar regulation and weight control. Limiting carbs with a high glycemic index during Phase One helps avoid sharp rises in blood sugar, which in turn lowers insulin secretion. This reduced insulin state promotes fat burning and reduces the desire for sweet foods.

Glycemic Control and Fat Storage: Eating foods with a low glycemic index is emphasized in the diet, which helps to stabilize blood sugar levels. Foods high in glucose frequently cause blood sugar levels to rise quickly, causing the body to release insulin, which can encourage the accumulation of fat. The diet reduces these spikes and encourages a more slow and regulated release of insulin by prioritizing low-glycemic meals, which encourages the use of fat for energy.

Impact on Hormonal Response: An important factor influencing hormonal response is the macronutrient balance of the South Beach Diet. Lean protein consumption aids in the control of hunger hormones, specifically leptin and ghrelin. Meals high in protein promote fullness and curb appetite by causing satiety and reducing hunger.

Function of Healthy Fats: The diet emphasizes the significance of healthy fats in controlling metabolism, dispelling the myth that all fats are bad. Without having an adverse effect on cholesterol levels, the monounsaturated and polyunsaturated fats present in avocados, nuts, seeds, and olive oil promote cellular health, facilitate nutrient absorption, and enhance feelings of fullness.

Metabolism and Muscle Preservation: A key component of the South Beach Diet is lean protein consumption for maintaining muscle mass. For metabolic health, it is essential to maintain a sufficient amount of muscle mass since muscle burns more calories at rest than fat. By emphasizing meals high in protein, the diet preserves muscle mass during weight loss and keeps the metabolic rate from dropping.

Nutrient Density and Health Benefits: The diet promotes foods high in nutrients, such as whole grains, fruits, and a range of vibrant vegetables. These foods are high in fiber, antioxidants, vitamins, and minerals, which enhance immune system function, lower the risk of chronic diseases, and provide vital nutrients for general health.

Evidence-Based Guidelines: Clinical studies and evidence-based research will serve as the foundation for the South Beach Diet's growth into 2024. The most recent scientific discoveries serve as the basis for ongoing diet updates and modifications, ensuring that dietary guidelines reflect the most recent advances in nutritional science.

The South Beach Diet's efficacy in maintaining muscle mass, managing insulin response, boosting metabolic health, and fostering better general health is supported by science. People can attain long-term health advantages and sustained weight management by following the diet's scientifically supported guidelines.

CHAPTER 7
Launching: Setting Up for Success

To achieve maximum success, starting the South Beach Diet involves careful planning and a calculated strategy. This chapter attempts to walk readers through the necessary preparations for starting the diet, developing a positive mindset, setting realistic goals, and setting up a setting that will support long-term adherence and fruitful results.

Knowing the Goals of the South Beach Diet: It's important to familiarize oneself with the goals and guiding principles of the South Beach Diet before starting. A strong foundation for success is created by comprehending the dietary requirements, the importance of macronutrient balance, the phased approach, and the reasoning behind the mechanics of the diet.

Evaluating Readiness and Commitment: It's critical to evaluate one's own readiness and level of commitment to changing one's diet. Setting reasonable expectations and coming up with solutions to problems are aided by thinking back on previous experiences, spotting possible difficulties, and assessing preparedness.

Setting Achievable and Specific Goals: Achieving goals that are specific, measurable, and unambiguous is essential to maintaining motivation and focus. Whether your goals are to improve your health markers, lose weight, or modify your lifestyle, SMART goals (Specific, Measurable, Achievable, Relevant, Time-bound) offer a path to success.

Planning and Preparation: The key to any diet's success is ahead of time planning. Making a grocery list of suggested meals, making sure the necessary items are available, and organizing a well-structured meal plan for the first few phases are important steps in eliminating impulsive purchases and encouraging adherence.

A supportive environment can be created by giving the kitchen a makeover, which includes getting rid of alluring but unhealthy meals and stocking up on staples that are permitted by the South Beach Diet. Maintaining a well-stocked pantry with nutrient-dense foods, whole grains, lean proteins, and healthy fats makes following a diet easier.

Education and Resources: Gaining the knowledge necessary to make wise judgments and comprehend the reasoning behind dietary choices can be achieved by educating oneself about the diet through trustworthy sources, such as respectable books, internet sites, or official South Beach Diet materials.

Accountability and Support System: Getting help from friends and family or joining a group of people who share your goals and objectives will help you stay motivated. A strong support network that allows for experience sharing, advice seeking, and achievement celebration is essential for maintaining adherence.

Embracing Flexibility and Patience: It's important to understand that adopting new food habits takes time and that lifestyle changes require patience. A positive outlook that is beneficial for long-term success is fostered by accepting flexibility, making allowances for sporadic errors, and engaging in self-compassion exercises in the face of failure.

More than simply food changes are needed to prepare for success on the South Beach Diet; a comprehensive strategy including goal-setting, planning, education, environment alteration, and a network of support is needed. People can position themselves for success and reach their health and weight management objectives by building a strong foundation and taking a proactive stance.

CHAPTER 8
Typical Fallacies and Misunderstandings

Like many popular diets, the South Beach Diet is subject to myths and misconceptions that are spread via hearsay, inaccurate information, or a misinterpretation of its guiding principles. This chapter seeks to clarify common misconceptions about the diet in order to provide readers with clarity and prevent them from accepting the diet's benefits to the fullest.

Myth number one:

"The South Beach Diet, is It A Low-Carb, No-Carb Diet"

Truth: The South Beach Diet is not a low-carb diet; rather, its initial phase limits high-glycemic-index carbs in an effort to balance blood sugar and encourage weight loss. To maintain weight loss and encourage a balanced diet, the later phases reintroduce healthy carbohydrates in moderation while highlighting whole grains, fruits, and certain vegetables.

The Second Myth:

"All Fats Are Forbidden on the South Beach Diet"

Reality: The diet promotes the consumption of beneficial fats while restricting the consumption of detrimental saturated and trans fats, debunking the myth that all fats are bad. Avocados, nuts, seeds, and olive oil include monounsaturated and polyunsaturated fats, which are essential for satiety, metabolic health, and general wellbeing.

Myth number three: "The South Beach Diet Is Only About Weight Loss"

Reality: Although losing weight is a major goal of the diet, other goals of the South Beach Diet as importance are improving general health and adopting sustainable lifestyles. Beyond just helping people lose extra weight, a balanced diet also attempts to improve metabolic parameters, control blood sugar, strengthen heart health, and increase general wellbeing.

Myth number four: "It's a Quick Fix or Short-Term Diet"

Reality: The South Beach Diet is meant to be a long-term lifestyle strategy, even if it promises quick weight loss during the initial phase. The structured approach promotes progressive and sustainable dietary improvements, highlighting the significance of continuous commitment to healthy eating practices and lifestyle adjustments for long-term success.

The fifth myth is that some foods must be expensive or specialized.

The South Beach Diet does not require specialty or pricey foods. It focuses mostly on whole, unprocessed foods that are easily found in most supermarkets. The majority of the foods that are advised are lean proteins, healthy fats, fruits, vegetables, and whole grains, making them both economical and readily available to most people.

Myth number six: "The Diet Lacks Sufficient Nutrients or Is Imbalanced"

Realization: The diet places a strong emphasis on nutrient-dense foods, guaranteeing a balanced consumption of vital vitamins, minerals, and antioxidants. The diet offers a balanced nutritional profile that supports general health and well-being by encouraging a range of vibrant vegetables, lean proteins, healthy fats, and whole grains.

Myth seven:

"The South Beach Diet Is One-Size-Fits-All"

Reality: The South Beach Diet is flexible enough to accommodate individual requirements and preferences, even though it provides organized recommendations. The diet recognizes individuality and permits changes to meal planning, serving sizes, and food selections according to personal objectives, dietary preferences, cultural factors, and medical concerns.

Making educated decisions and putting the South Beach Diet into practice need knowing the truths underlying the widespread myths and misconceptions about it. People can accept the diet's tenets, appreciate its flexibility, and take advantage of its efficacy in reaching long-term health and weight control objectives by busting these misconceptions.

CHAPTER 9
Success Strategies and Long-Term Outcomes

Dedication, persistence, and a calculated approach are necessary to succeed in the South Beach Diet and sustain long-term outcomes. This chapter offers detailed advice on how to improve compliance, cultivate good habits, overcome obstacles, and maintain the diet's benefits for long-term health and wellbeing.

First tip: Adopt a Phased Approach

Acknowledge the significance of every stage and follow the instructions given. Phase One expedites the loss of weight, Phase Two reintroduces nutritious carbohydrates, and Phase Three concentrates on maintenance. Observe the suggested diet, respect the progression, and move between phases with awareness.

Tip 2: Arrange and Prepare Meals: A successful meal plan is essential. Create a weekly meal plan that follows the guidelines of the South Beach Diet. To ensure adherence to dietary rules and prevent impulsive decisions, prepare meals ahead of time. Preparing and cooking materials in bulk can streamline compliance and save time.

Tip 3: Eat in Moderation:

Portion sizes matter, even when eating healthful meals. Utilize visual cues or measurement devices to determine the proper portion sizes. Even while eating healthily, overindulging can impede the process of losing weight. Maintaining long-term success is facilitated by learning portion control.

Tip 4: Drink Plenty of Water:

Water is essential for both general health and weight loss. Make it a point to stay hydrated during the day by drinking enough water. Maintaining hydration promotes metabolic processes, reduces appetite, and facilitates digestion.

Tip 5: Include Physical Activity:

For best outcomes, combine nutrition and regular exercise. Take part in something you enjoy doing; it could be yoga, strength training, walking, or running. Engaging in physical activity enhances weight loss and promotes general health and wellbeing.

Tip 6: Mindful Eating Practices:

Slow down, pay attention to your hunger, and enjoy every mouthful of food as you practice mindful eating. To improve your relationship with food and avoid overindulging, keep your mind off of other things while you eat, such as watching TV or using electronic gadgets.

Tip 7: Seek Accountability and Support:

Participate in online groups, join a support group, or look for friends or family who are embarking on a similar diet. Having a network of support provides inspiration, responsibility, and a forum for exchanging advice and experiences.

Tip 8: Learn from Setbacks:

Accept that obstacles will arise along the way. If you commit an error, get past it. Rather, assess the circumstance, pinpoint the causes, and make use of it as a teaching moment. In order to avoid more defeats, review objectives and tactics and make necessary adjustments.

Tip 9: Honor Non-Scale Achievements:

Celebrate and acknowledge accomplishments that go above and beyond. Gains include more vitality, restful sleep, heightened endurance, and more fit in clothes. Acknowledging these non-scale successes can improve morale and motivation.

Tip 10: Develop a Sustainable Mentality

Accept the South Beach Diet as a way of life rather than a short-term solution. Put your attention on developing wholesome routines and a well-rounded eating style. Aim for long-term health and well-being and strive for development rather than perfection.

The South Beach Diet requires a combination of calculated methods, constant adherence, a positive outlook, and continuous dedication to good habits in order to be successful. People can attain long-term success, maintain short-term goals, and enjoy the advantages of better health and long-term weight management by adopting these suggestions into their everyday routines.

CHAPTER 10
Frequently Asked Questions (FAQs)

1. Describe the South Beach Diet and its methodology.

The South Beach Diet is a well-liked weight-reduction and health-improvement plan created to control blood sugar levels, encourage wholesome eating, and provide long-term weight loss. It works in three stages: Phase One involves cutting out processed carbohydrates and sugars; Phase Two involves progressively reintroducing healthy carbohydrates; and Phase Three concentrates on keeping a balanced diet.

2. Is everyone a good fit for the South Beach Diet?

For the majority of people, the diet is suitable. Before beginning any new diet, it is best to speak with a healthcare provider, especially if you have any pre-existing medical conditions or are pregnant or breastfeeding a baby.

3. What kind of food is allowed on the South Beach Diet?

Lean proteins, good fats, whole grains, fruits, vegetables, and low-fat dairy products are the mainstays of the diet. Fish, poultry, eggs, nuts, seeds, olive oil, whole grains, legumes, and an array of vibrant fruits and vegetables are among the foods that are advised.

4. *Is there a low-carb version of the South Beach Diet?*

Although the first phase limits carbohydrates with a high glycemic index, the diet is not strictly low-carb. It centers on regulating the caliber of carbs ingested, with a gradual return to healthier options in subsequent stages.

5. *On the South Beach Diet, how much weight can I hope to lose?*

Individual differences in weight loss are attributed to various factors, including initial weight, diet compliance, and degree of physical activity. Because of decreased water retention and fat burning during the first phase, quick weight reduction is typical, with sustained progress occurring throughout subsequent phases.

6. *Can a vegetarian or vegan follow the South Beach Diet?*

It is possible to adjust the diet to accommodate vegetarian or vegan preferences by changing the sources of protein. Dietary needs can be met by including a range of vegetables and whole grains, beans, tofu, and tempeh, among other plant-based proteins.

7. How long should I adhere to each South Beach Diet phase?

Every phase has a different time based on personal preferences, weight loss ambitions, and individual goals. Phase One usually lasts for two weeks, Phase Two continues until weight objectives are met, and Phase Three focuses on maintaining weight and forming healthy behaviors for the rest of one's life.

8. Is alcohol allowed while following the South Beach Diet?

It is not recommended to consume alcohol during the beginning phases of the program as it may impede weight loss efforts. Moderation is crucial when it comes to alcohol use, and selecting lower-carb options such as dry wines or spirits with low-calorie mixers is advised.

9. What should I do if I hit a weight-loss wall?

Plateaus in weight loss are typical. If you reach a plateau, evaluate how closely you're following the diet instructions, take a second look at portion sizes, up your physical activity level, and think about getting advice from a dietician or medical specialist.

10. How can I keep losing weight once the South Beach Diet is over?

Keep in mind the healthy behaviors you developed on the diet: proceed with mindful eating, portion management, frequent exercise, and balanced meals. Regular weight monitoring, getting help, and adopting a long-term mindset about health are crucial.

The FAQs for the South Beach Diet provide insightful answers to frequently asked questions concerning the diet's tenets, acceptable foods, suitability, anticipated weight reduction, sustainability, and long-term success tactics. People can effectively navigate the diet, make educated decisions, and accomplish their health and weight management objectives by being aware of these FAQs.

PART TWO
Part Two: Practical Implementation and Meal Plans

Phase One: Reset Your Body

<u>**Give Your Body a Break**</u>

<u>**Overview and Guidelines for Phase One**</u>

The South Beach Diet's first phase is the cornerstone for resetting your body and accelerating weight reduction. An outline of the rules is provided below:

Goals: Lower blood sugar, lessen sugar and refined carbohydrate cravings, and start losing weight quickly.

Length: Usually, this stage takes two weeks.

<u>**Important Rules:**</u>

Food Focus: Low-glycemic index meals, healthy fats, high-fiber veggies, and lean proteins.

Foods to Steer Clear of: fruits, starchy vegetables, refined sugars, and processed carbs.

Meal Structure: To guarantee fullness and blood sugar stability, eat three balanced meals and snacks each day.

Portion Control: To avoid overindulging, place a focus on sensible portion proportions.

Hydration: Drinking enough water can boost metabolism and reduce cravings.

Phase One Meal Plan Structure
Phase One Meal Recipes

Breakfast Recipes

Vegetable Omelet

Preparation time: 10 minutes

Cooking time: 10 minutes

Total time: 20 minutes

Servings: 1

Ingredients:

- 2 eggs
- 1/4 cup chopped bell peppers
- 1/4 cup chopped onions
- 1/4 cup chopped spinach
- 1/4 cup crumbled feta cheese
- Salt and pepper to taste
- 1 tablespoon olive oil

Directions:

- ➤ Mix the eggs together with the salt and pepper in a bowl.
- ➤ In a nonstick skillet, warm the olive oil over medium heat.
- ➤ Add the bell peppers and onions and sauté for 2-3 minutes until softened.
- ➤ Add the spinach and sauté for another minute until wilted.
- ➤ Pour the eggs over the vegetables and cook until set, about 3-4 minutes.
- ➤ Sprinkle the feta cheese over the omelet and fold it in half.
- ➤ Cook for another minute or so, or until the cheese melts.
- ➤ Serve hot.

Greek Yogurt with Berries

Preparation time: 5 minutes

Total time: 5 minutes

Servings: 1

Ingredients:

- 1/2 cup plain Greek yogurt
- 1/4 cup mixed berries (such as blueberries, raspberries, and strawberries)
- 1 tablespoon chopped nuts (such as almonds or walnuts)

Directions:

- ➢ In a bowl, mix the Greek yogurt with the chopped nuts.
- ➢ Top with the mixed berries.
- ➢ Serve chilled.

Crustless Quiche

Preparation time: 10 minutes

Cooking time: 30 minutes

Total time: 40 minutes

Servings: 4

Ingredients:

- 6 eggs
- 1 cup chopped spinach
- 1/2 cup chopped mushrooms
- 1/4 cup crumbled feta cheese
- Salt and pepper to taste
- 1 tablespoon olive oil

Directions:

➢ Preheat the oven to 350°F.
➢ Combine the eggs along with the salt and pepper in a bowl.
➢ In a nonstick skillet, warm the olive oil over medium heat.
➢ Add the spinach and mushrooms and sauté for 2-3 minutes until softened.
➢ Pour the eggs over the vegetables and sprinkle the feta cheese on top.
➢ Bake in the preheated oven for 25-30 minutes until set and golden.
➢ Before slicing, let it chill for a few minutes.
➢ Serve warm.

Turkey and Egg Breakfast Casserole

Preparation time: 10 minutes

Cooking time: 30 minutes

Total time: 40 minutes

Servings: 4

Ingredients:

- 1 pound ground turkey
- 6 eggs
- 1/2 cup chopped bell peppers
- 1/2 cup chopped onions
- Salt and pepper to taste
- 1 tablespoon olive oil

Directions:

➢ Preheat the oven to 350°F.

➢ In a nonstick skillet, warm the olive oil over medium heat.

➢ Add the ground turkey and sauté for 5-7 minutes until browned.

➢ Add the bell peppers and onions and sauté for 2-3 minutes until softened.

➢ Mix the eggs along with the salt and pepper in a bowl.

- ➢ Grease a baking dish with cooking spray.
- ➢ Spread the turkey mixture evenly in the baking dish.
- ➢ Pour the eggs over the turkey mixture.
- ➢ Bake in the preheated oven for 25-30 minutes until set and golden.
- ➢ Before slicing, let it cool for a few minutes.
- ➢ Serve warm.

Ricotta and Cinnamon Pancakes

Preparation time: 10 minutes

Cooking time: 10 minutes

Total time: 20 minutes

Servings: 2

Ingredients:

- 1/2 cup ricotta cheese
- 2 eggs
- 1/2 teaspoon ground cinnamon
- 1/2 teaspoon vanilla extract
- 1/4 teaspoon baking powder
- Salt to taste
- Cooking spray

Directions:

- ➢ In a bowl, whisk the ricotta cheese, eggs, cinnamon, vanilla extract, baking powder, and salt until smooth.
- ➢ A nonstick skillet should be heated to medium heat.
- ➢ Grease the skillet with cooking spray.
- ➢ For each pancake, pour a quarter-cup of the batter into the skillet.
- ➢ Simmer for two to three minutes, or until surface bubbles appear.
- ➢ After flipping, cook for a further minute or until golden.
- ➢ Repeat with the remaining batter.
- ➢ Serve hot with sugar-free syrup.

Egg and Vegetable Muffins

Preparation time: 10 minutes

Cooking time: 20 minutes

Total time: 30 minutes

Servings: 6

Ingredients:

- 6 eggs
- 1/2 cup chopped spinach
- 1/2 cup chopped tomatoes
- 1/4 cup chopped bell peppers
- Salt and pepper to taste
- Cooking spray

Directions:

➢ Preheat the oven to 350°F.
➢ Grease a muffin tin with cooking spray.
➢ Whisk the eggs along with the salt and pepper in a bowl.
➢ Add the chopped vegetables and mix well.
➢ Spoon the egg mixture into each muffin tray, filling it to about three-quarters of the way.
➢ Bake for 15 to 20 minutes, or until firm and brown, in a preheated oven.
➢ Let cool for a few minutes before removing from the muffin tin.
➢ Serve warm.

Smoked Salmon Roll-Ups

Preparation time: 10 minutes

Total time: 10 minutes

Servings: 2

Ingredients:

- 4 slices smoked salmon
- 2 tablespoons cream cheese
- 4 cucumber slices

Directions:

➤ Lay the smoked salmon slices on a cutting board.

➤ Spread the cream cheese on the salmon slices.

➤ Place a cucumber slice on each salmon slice.

➤ Roll up the salmon slices.

➤ Serve chilled.

Avocado and Egg Salad

Preparation time: 10 minutes

Total time: 10 minutes

Servings: 2

Ingredients:

- 4 hard-boiled eggs, chopped
- 1 avocado, chopped
- 1/2 cup cherry tomatoes, halved
- 2 cups lettuce
- Salt and pepper to taste
- 1 tablespoon olive oil

Directions:

- ➢ In a bowl, mix the chopped eggs, avocado, and cherry tomatoes.
- ➢ Add the lettuce and mix well.
- ➢ Drizzle the olive oil over the salad.
- ➢ Season with salt and pepper to taste

Cottage Cheese and Almond Bowl

Preparation time: 5 minutes

Total time: 5 minutes

Servings: 1

Ingredients:

- 1 cup cottage cheese
- 1/4 cup almonds, chopped
- 1 tablespoon honey
- 1/2 teaspoon vanilla extract
- 1/4 teaspoon cinnamon
- Fruit of your choice (such as berries, sliced almonds, or mango)

Directions:

- In a bowl, mix the cottage cheese, almonds, honey, vanilla extract, and cinnamon until smooth.
- Serve the cottage cheese mixture in a glass or bowl.
- Top with your choice of fruit and additional almonds.
- Drizzle with honey and sprinkle with cinnamon.

Chia Seed Pudding

Preparation time: 10 minutes

Cooking time: 2 hours

Total time: 2 hours and 10 minutes

Servings: 4

Ingredients:

- 1/4 cup chia seeds
- 1 1/2 cups unsweetened almond milk
- 1 tablespoon maple syrup or honey
- 1 teaspoon vanilla extract
- Pinch of salt
- Optional toppings: fresh berries, nuts, or seeds

Directions:

- ➢ In a bowl or mason jar, combine the chia seeds, almond milk, maple syrup, vanilla extract, and salt.
- ➢ Mix well and let the mixture sit for 2 hours or overnight in the refrigerator.
- ➢ Stir the pudding every 30 minutes during the initial 2 hours to ensure the chia seeds are fully hydrated.
- ➢ After 2 hours, the pudding should have thickened and set up.
- ➢ Serve chilled with your choice of toppings, such as fresh berries, nuts, or seeds.

Grilled Chicken Salad

Preparation Time: 20 minutes

Cooking Time: 10 minutes

Total Time: 30 minutes

Servings: 4

Ingredients:

- 1 lb boneless, skinless chicken breasts
- 1 tablespoon olive oil
- Salt and pepper to taste
- 6 cups mixed salad greens
- 1 cup cherry tomatoes, halved
- 1 cucumber, sliced
- 1/2 red onion, thinly sliced
- 1/4 cup feta cheese, crumbled
- Dressing of your choice (balsamic vinaigrette or ranch work well)

Directions:

- ➢ Preheat the grill to medium-high heat.
- ➢ Add salt and pepper to the chicken breasts after brushing them with olive oil.

- ➤ Grill the chicken for about 4-5 minutes per side or until fully cooked through (internal temperature of 165°F or 74°C). Before slicing, let it a few minutes to rest.
- ➤ Mix the cucumber, red onion, cherry tomatoes, and salad leaves in a big bowl.
- ➤ Slice the grilled chicken breasts and place them on top of the salad.
- ➤ Sprinkle crumbled feta cheese over the salad.
- ➤ Drizzle your preferred dressing over the salad and toss gently to combine.
- ➤ Serve immediately and enjoy your flavorful grilled chicken salad!

Tuna Lettuce Wraps

Preparation Time: 15 minutes

Total Time: 15 minutes

Servings: 2-3

Ingredients:

- 2 cans (5 oz each) tuna, drained
- 1/4 cup mayonnaise
- 2 tablespoons chopped celery
- 2 tablespoons chopped red onion
- 1 tablespoon lemon juice
- Salt and pepper to taste
- 6 large lettuce leaves (butter lettuce or iceberg lettuce work well)
- Optional: Avocado slices, diced tomatoes, or cucumber slices for garnish

Directions:

- ➤ In a mixing bowl, combine the drained tuna, mayonnaise, chopped celery, chopped red onion, and lemon juice. Season with salt and pepper. Mix well.
- ➤ Place a spoonful of the tuna mixture onto each lettuce leaf.

➢ Add optional garnishes like avocado slices, diced tomatoes, or cucumber slices if desired.

➢ Roll up the lettuce leaves with the tuna mixture inside, securing them with toothpicks if needed.

➢ Arrange the lettuce wraps on a serving platter and serve immediately.

Eggplant and Mozzarella Stacks

Preparation Time: 15 minutes

Cooking Time: 20 minutes

Total Time: 35 minutes

Servings: 2

Ingredients:

- One large eggplant cut into rounds, each about half an inch thick
- 2 medium tomatoes, sliced
- 8 oz fresh mozzarella cheese, sliced
- 1/4 cup fresh basil leaves
- Balsamic glaze (store-bought or homemade)
- Olive oil
- Salt and pepper to taste

Directions:

➢ Preheat the oven to 400°F (200°C).

➢ Add salt and pepper to the eggplant slices after brushing them with olive oil on both sides.

➢ Place the eggplant slices on a baking sheet and bake for 10-12 minutes, flipping halfway through, until they are tender and lightly golden.

➢ Remove the eggplant slices from the oven and let them cool slightly.

➢ Assemble the stacks by layering the eggplant slices, tomato slices, mozzarella slices, and fresh basil leaves, repeating until you have stacks about 2-3 layers high.

➢ Drizzle each stack with balsamic glaze.

➢ Place the stacks back in the oven for an additional 5-8 minutes or until the cheese is melted and bubbly.

➢ Serve warm as a delightful appetizer or main course.

Turkey and Avocado Roll-Ups

Preparation Time: 10 minutes

Total Time: 10 minutes

Servings: 4

Ingredients:

- 8 slices deli turkey
- 1 ripe avocado, sliced
- 1/2 red bell pepper, thinly sliced
- 1 cup baby spinach leaves
- 1 tablespoon cream cheese (optional)
- Toothpicks

Directions:

- ➢ Lay out the turkey slices on a clean surface.
- ➢ Spread a thin layer of cream cheese (if using) onto each turkey slice.
- ➢ Place a few spinach leaves on top of each turkey slice.
- ➢ Add avocado slices and red bell pepper strips on one end of each turkey slice.
- ➢ Carefully roll up each slice, starting from the end with the fillings, and secure with toothpicks to keep them in place.
- ➢ Arrange the roll-ups on a serving plate and serve as a delicious and healthy snack or light lunch option.

Salmon and Asparagus Foil Packs

Preparation Time: 10 minutes

Cooking Time: 20 minutes

Total Time: 30 minutes

Servings: 2

Ingredients:

- 2 salmon fillets (6 oz each)
- 1 bunch asparagus, trimmed
- 2 cloves garlic, minced
- 2 tablespoons olive oil
- 1 tablespoon lemon juice
- Salt and pepper to taste
- Fresh dill or parsley for garnish

Directions:

➢ Preheat the oven to 400°F (200°C).

➢ Cut two large pieces of aluminum foil.

➢ Place half of the asparagus spears in the center of each piece of foil.

➢ Season the salmon fillets with salt, pepper, minced garlic, olive oil, and lemon juice. Place one fillet on top of the bed of asparagus on each foil piece.

➢ Fold the sides of the foil over the salmon and asparagus, sealing the edges tightly to create a packet.

➢ Place the foil packs on a baking sheet and bake in the preheated oven for about 15-20 minutes, or until the salmon is cooked through and flakes easily with a fork.

➢ Carefully open the foil packs, garnish with fresh dill or parsley, and serve hot.

Cauliflower Rice Sushi Rolls

Preparation Time: 30 minutes

Cooking Time: 10 minutes

Total Time: 40 minutes

Servings: 4

Ingredients:

- 1 head cauliflower
- 2 tablespoons rice vinegar
- 1 tablespoon sugar
- Salt to taste
- 4 sheets nori seaweed
- Assorted fillings (cucumber sticks, avocado slices, imitation crab sticks, etc.)
- For serving, add wasabi, pickled ginger, and soy sauce (optional).

Directions:

- In a food processor, pulse the cauliflower until it resembles rice after cutting it into florets.
- In a skillet, heat a tablespoon of oil over medium heat. Cook the cauliflower rice for five to seven minutes, or until it becomes soft.

- In a small bowl, mix the sugar, salt, and rice vinegar. Stir this mixture into the cooked cauliflower rice and let it cool.
- Lay down a nori sheet on a fresh kitchen towel or a bamboo sushi mat.
- Spread an even layer of cauliflower rice over the nori, leaving a small border at the top.
- Add your desired fillings in a row along the bottom edge of the nori.
- Roll the sushi tightly using the bamboo mat or towel, sealing the edge with a little water.
- Repeat the process with the remaining nori sheets and fillings.
- Slice the rolls into bite-sized pieces using a sharp knife.
- Serve the cauliflower rice sushi rolls with soy sauce, pickled ginger, and wasabi if desired.

Mediterranean Tuna Salad

Preparation Time: 15 minutes

Total Time: 15 minutes

Servings: 2-3

Ingredients:

- 2 cans (5 oz each) tuna, drained
- 1/2 cup cherry tomatoes, halved
- 1/2 cucumber, diced
- 1/4 cup red onion, finely chopped
- 1/4 cup Kalamata olives, sliced
- 2 tablespoons chopped fresh parsley
- 2 tablespoons olive oil
- 1 tablespoon lemon juice
- Salt and pepper to taste
- Mixed salad greens or lettuce leaves for serving

Directions:

➢ In a mixing bowl, combine the drained tuna, cherry tomatoes, cucumber, red onion, Kalamata olives, and chopped parsley.
➢ Drizzle olive oil and lemon juice over the tuna mixture.
➢ Add salt and pepper to taste, and toss lightly to mix.
➢ Serve the Mediterranean tuna salad over a bed of mixed salad greens or lettuce leaves.

Chicken and Vegetable Skewers

Preparation Time: 20 minutes

Cooking Time: 10 minutes

Total Time: 30 minutes

Servings: 4

Ingredients:

- One pound of chopped, skinless, and boneless chicken breasts
- 1 red bell pepper, cut into chunks
- 1 yellow bell pepper, cut into chunks
- 1 red onion, cut into chunks
- 8-10 cherry tomatoes
- 1 zucchini, sliced
- 2 tablespoons olive oil
- 2 cloves garlic, minced
- 1 teaspoon paprika
- Salt and pepper to taste
- 30 minutes of soaking time for wooden skewers

Directions:

- Turn the heat up to medium-high on the grill or grill pan.

- Mix the paprika, olive oil, minced garlic, salt, and pepper in a bowl.
- Thread the chicken, bell peppers, onion, cherry tomatoes, and zucchini onto the soaked skewers, alternating the ingredients.
- Brush the skewers with the prepared olive oil mixture.
- Grill the skewers for about 4-5 minutes per side or until the chicken is fully cooked and the vegetables are tender.
- Remove the skewers from the grill and serve hot.

Zucchini Noodles with Pesto and Cherry Tomatoes

Preparation Time: 15 minutes

Cooking Time: 5 minutes

Total Time: 20 minutes

Servings: 2-3

Ingredients:

- 3 medium zucchinis, spiralized into noodles
- 1 cup cherry tomatoes, halved
- 1/4 cup prepared pesto sauce
- 2 tablespoons grated Parmesan cheese
- Salt and pepper to taste
- Olive oil for cooking

Directions:

➢ One tablespoon of olive oil should be heated over medium heat in a skillet.

➢ Add the zucchini noodles and cherry tomatoes to the skillet. Sauté for 3-4 minutes until the noodles are slightly softened but still tender-crisp.

➢ Stir in the pesto sauce and cook for an additional minute until heated through.

- ➤ Season with salt and pepper to taste.
- ➤ Remove from heat and sprinkle grated Parmesan cheese over the zucchini noodles.
- ➤ Serve immediately as a delicious low-carb alternative to pasta.

Turkey and Spinach Stuffed Mushrooms

Preparation Time: 20 minutes

Cooking Time: 25 minutes

Total Time: 45 minutes

Servings: 4

Ingredients:

- 16 large mushrooms, stems removed and reserved
- 1/2 lb ground turkey
- 1/2 onion, finely chopped
- 2 cloves garlic, minced
- 1 cup fresh spinach, chopped
- 1/4 cup breadcrumbs
- 1/4 cup grated Parmesan cheese
- 2 tablespoons olive oil
- Salt and pepper to taste
- Fresh parsley for garnish

Directions:

➢ Preheat the oven to 375°F (190°C).

- Chop the mushroom stems finely.
- In an iron skillet over a medium-high flame, warm the olive oil. Add chopped mushroom stems, onion, and garlic. Sauté until softened.
- Cook the ground turkey in the skillet until it is browned. Season with salt and pepper.
- Stir in the chopped spinach and cook until wilted. Remove from heat.
- In a bowl, combine the turkey mixture with breadcrumbs and grated Parmesan cheese.
- Spoon the turkey mixture into the mushroom caps, filling each generously.
- After placing the filled mushrooms on a baking sheet, bake them for 20 to 25 minutes, or until the filling is golden brown and the mushrooms are soft
- Garnish with fresh parsley before serving.

These recipes offer a variety of delicious and healthy lunch options. Enjoy preparing and savoring these meals!

Baked Lemon Herb Chicken

Preparation Time: 10 minutes

Cooking Time: 25-30 minutes

Total Time: 35-40 minutes

Servings: 4

Ingredients:

- 4 boneless, skinless chicken breasts
- 2 tablespoons olive oil
- Zest of 1 lemon
- Juice of 1 lemon
- 2 cloves garlic, minced
- 1 teaspoon dried oregano
- 1 teaspoon dried thyme
- Salt and pepper to taste
- Fresh parsley for garnish (optional)

Directions:

➢ Preheat the oven to 400°F (200°C). Grease a baking dish with olive oil or line it with parchment paper.

- In a small bowl, mix together olive oil, lemon zest, lemon juice, minced garlic, dried oregano, dried thyme, salt, and pepper.
- Pat the chicken breasts dry with paper towels and place them in the prepared baking dish.
- Brush the lemon herb mixture over the chicken breasts, ensuring they are evenly coated.
- Bake the chicken for 25 to 30 minutes, or until its internal temperature reaches 165°F (74°C), in a preheated oven.
- Once done, remove from the oven and let the chicken rest for a few minutes before serving.
- Garnish with fresh parsley if desired and serve the flavorful baked lemon herb chicken.

Cauliflower Rice Stir-Fry

Preparation Time: 15 minutes

Cooking Time: 15 minutes

Total Time: 30 minutes

Servings: 4

Ingredients:

- 1 head cauliflower
- 2 tablespoons sesame oil or olive oil
- 2 cloves garlic, minced
- 1 small onion, diced
- 1 cup mixed vegetables (bell peppers, carrots, peas, etc.), chopped
- 3 tablespoons low-sodium soy sauce or tamari
- 2 eggs, beaten (optional)
- Salt and pepper to taste
- Green onions for garnish

Directions:

➢ Wash the cauliflower and cut it into florets. In a food processor, pulse the florets until they have the texture of rice grains.

- Heat sesame oil or olive oil in a large skillet or wok over medium-high heat.
- Add minced garlic and diced onion, sauté for 2-3 minutes until fragrant.
- Add the chopped mixed vegetables to the skillet and stir-fry for about 3-4 minutes until they start to soften.
- Push the vegetables to one side of the skillet and pour the beaten eggs (if using) onto the empty side. After the eggs are cooked, scramble them and combine them with the vegetables.
- Add the cauliflower rice to the skillet and stir-fry for 4-5 minutes until it's cooked but still slightly crisp.
- Pour soy sauce or tamari over the cauliflower rice and mix well.
- To taste, add salt and pepper for seasoning.
- Garnish with chopped green onions before serving this delicious cauliflower rice stir-fry.

Shrimp and Zucchini Noodles

Preparation Time: 15 minutes

Cooking Time: 10 minutes

Total Time: 25 minutes

Servings: 2

Ingredients:

- 2 medium zucchinis, spiralized into noodles
- 12-16 large shrimp, peeled and deveined
- 2 tablespoons olive oil
- 3 cloves garlic, minced
- 1/4 teaspoon red pepper flakes (optional)
- Juice of 1/2 lemon
- Salt and pepper to taste
- Chopped fresh parsley for garnish

Directions:

➢ In a big skillet over medium heat, warm up the olive oil.

➢ Add red pepper flakes (if using) and minced garlic to the skillet. Sauté until aromatic, about 30 seconds.

➢ When the shrimp are pink and opaque, add them to the skillet and cook for two to three minutes on each side. Remove the shrimp from the skillet and set aside.

- In the same skillet, add the spiralized zucchini noodles and lemon juice. Sauté for 2-3 minutes until the noodles are just tender but still have a slight crunch.
- Add a little salt and pepper to the zucchini noodles.
- Return the cooked shrimp to the skillet and toss everything together for a minute to heat through.
- Garnish with chopped fresh parsley before serving these delightful shrimp and zucchini noodles.

Turkey and Spinach Meatballs

Preparation Time: 15 minutes

Cooking Time: 20 minutes

Total Time: 35 minutes

Servings: 4

Ingredients:

- 1 lb ground turkey
- 1/2 cup breadcrumbs
- 1/4 cup grated Parmesan cheese
- 1/4 cup chopped fresh parsley
- 1/4 cup chopped fresh spinach
- 1 egg
- 2 cloves garlic, minced
- 1 teaspoon dried oregano
- 1/2 teaspoon onion powder
- Salt and pepper to taste
- Olive oil for cooking

Directions:

➢ Preheat the oven to 375°F (190°C). Use parchment paper to line a baking sheet.

- In a large mixing bowl, combine ground turkey, breadcrumbs, grated Parmesan cheese, chopped parsley, chopped spinach, egg, minced garlic, dried oregano, onion powder, salt, and pepper. Mix until well combined.
- Shape the mixture into meatballs, about 1-2 inches in diameter, and place them on the prepared baking sheet.
- Drizzle or brush the meatballs lightly with olive oil.
- Bake in the preheated oven for 18-20 minutes or until the meatballs are cooked through and golden brown.
- Serve these flavorful turkey and spinach meatballs on their own or with your favorite sauce.

Grilled Steak with Roasted Vegetables

Preparation Time: 15 minutes

Cooking Time: 20 minutes

Total Time: 35 minutes

Servings: 2

Ingredients:

- Two steaks, cut to your preference (sirloin, ribeye, etc.)
- 2 tablespoons olive oil
- 2 cloves garlic, minced
- 1 teaspoon dried rosemary
- 1 teaspoon dried thyme
- Salt and pepper to taste
- Assorted vegetables (bell peppers, carrots, zucchini, etc.), cut into chunks for roasting
- Fresh herbs for garnish (optional)

Directions:

➢ Preheat the grill to medium-high heat.

➢ Rub the steaks with olive oil, minced garlic, dried rosemary, dried thyme, salt, and pepper. Ensure the steaks are evenly coated with the seasoning.

- ➢ Grill the steaks for 4-6 minutes per side, depending on the desired level of doneness.
- ➢ While the steaks are grilling, toss the assorted vegetables with olive oil, salt, and pepper.
- ➢ Place the seasoned vegetables on a baking sheet and roast them in the oven at 400°F (200°C) for 15-20 minutes or until they are tender and lightly browned.
- ➢ Before slicing, take the steaks off the grill and let them a few minutes to rest.
- ➢ Serve the grilled steak slices with the roasted vegetables and garnish with fresh herbs if desired.

Baked Cod with Lemon and Dill

Preparation Time: 10 minutes

Cooking Time: 15 minutes

Total Time: 25 minutes

Servings: 2

Ingredients:

- 2 cod fillets (6-8 oz each)
- 2 tablespoons melted butter or olive oil
- Juice of 1 lemon
- 2 cloves garlic, minced
- 1 tablespoon chopped fresh dill (or 1 teaspoon dried dill)
- Salt and pepper to taste
- Lemon slices for garnish

Directions:

➢ Preheat the oven to 400°F (200°C). Grease a baking dish with oil or butter.

➢ Pat the cod fillets dry with paper towels and place them in the prepared baking dish.

➢ In a small bowl, mix together melted butter or olive oil, lemon juice, minced garlic, chopped dill, salt, and pepper.

- Pour the lemon-dill mixture over the cod fillets, ensuring they are evenly coated.
- Place lemon slices on top of each fillet for added flavor and moisture.
- Bake in the preheated oven for 12-15 minutes or until the fish flakes easily with a fork and is opaque throughout.
- Serve the baked cod with additional lemon wedges if desired.

Eggplant Lasagna

Preparation Time: 30 minutes

Cooking Time: 45 minutes

Total Time: 1 hour 15 minutes

Servings: 6

Ingredients:

- 2 medium eggplants, sliced lengthwise into 1/4-inch thick slices
- 2 cups marinara sauce
- 1 lb ground beef or turkey (optional)
- 2 cups ricotta cheese
- 1 cup shredded mozzarella cheese
- 1/2 cup grated Parmesan cheese
- 2 cloves garlic, minced
- 1 tablespoon olive oil
- 1 teaspoon dried basil
- 1 teaspoon dried oregano
- Salt and pepper to taste
- Fresh basil leaves for garnish (optional)

Directions:

- Preheat the oven to 375°F (190°C). Grease a baking dish with olive oil.
- Place eggplant slices on a baking sheet. Sprinkle them with salt and let them sit for about 15 minutes to draw out excess moisture. Pat dry with paper towels.
- In a skillet, heat olive oil over medium heat. Add the minced garlic and cook it for a few seconds, until it becomes aromatic.
- If using ground meat, add it to the skillet and cook until browned. Drain excess fat.
- Stir in marinara sauce, dried basil, dried oregano, salt, and pepper. Simmer for a few minutes.
- Apply a thin coating of the meat sauce to the baking dish that has been buttered.
- Arrange a layer of eggplant slices over the sauce, followed by a layer of ricotta cheese, mozzarella cheese, and Parmesan cheese. Repeat the layers, finishing with a final layer of sauce and cheese on top.
- Bake the dish for thirty minutes with the foil covering it. After 15 more minutes of baking, take off the foil and continue baking until the cheese turns golden and bubbling.
- Let it cool for a few minutes before slicing. Garnish with fresh basil leaves if desired and serve this delectable eggplant lasagna.

Cabbage and Beef Stir-Fry

Preparation Time: 15 minutes

Cooking Time: 15 minutes

Total Time: 30 minutes

Servings: 4

Ingredients:

- 1 lb ground beef
- 1 small cabbage, thinly sliced
- 1 onion, thinly sliced
- 2 cloves garlic, minced
- 2 tablespoons soy sauce
- 1 tablespoon sesame oil
- 1 tablespoon rice vinegar
- 1 teaspoon ginger, minced
- 1 teaspoon Sriracha sauce (optional)
- Salt and pepper to taste
- Green onions for garnish (optional)

Directions:

In a bowl, mix together soy sauce, sesame oil, rice vinegar, minced ginger, and Sriracha sauce (if using). Set aside.

In a big skillet or wok, heat up one tablespoon of oil over medium-high heat.

To the skillet, add the onion slices and minced garlic. Sauté for about 2 minutes until fragrant.

Using a spatula, break up the ground beef while it cooks until it turns brown.

Add the thinly sliced cabbage to the skillet and stir-fry for 4-5 minutes until it starts to wilt but remains slightly crunchy.

Pour the prepared sauce over the beef and cabbage mixture. Coat everything with the sauce by giving everything a good stir.

Season with salt and pepper to taste.

Cook for a further two to three minutes, or until well heated.

Garnish with chopped green onions if desired before serving this flavorful cabbage and beef stir-fry.

Zucchini Boats with Ground Turkey

Preparation time: 15 minutes

Cooking time: 30 minutes

Total time: 45 minutes

Servings: 4

Ingredients:

- 4 medium zucchinis, halved lengthwise
- 1 pound ground turkey
- 1/2 cup chopped onions
- 2 cloves garlic, minced
- 1/2 cup marinara sauce
- 1/2 cup shredded mozzarella cheese
- 2 tablespoons olive oil
- Salt and pepper to taste

Directions:

- ➢ Preheat the oven to 375°F.
- ➢ Scoop out the flesh of the zucchinis with a spoon, leaving a 1/4-inch border around the edges.
- ➢ In a bowl, mix together the ground turkey, onions, garlic, salt, and pepper until well combined.

- The olive oil should be warmed over medium heat in a large skillet.
- Add the ground turkey mixture and sauté for 5-7 minutes until browned.
- Add the marinara sauce and cook for another 2-3 minutes until heated through.
- Fill the zucchini boats with spoonfuls of the turkey mixture.
- Over the turkey mixture, scatter the mozzarella cheese shreds.
- Bake in the preheated oven for 20-25 minutes until the zucchinis are tender and the cheese is melted and golden.
- Let cool for a few minutes before serving

Phase One Meal Plan Structure

Here's a two-week meal plan structure incorporating the provided Phase One recipes for breakfast, lunch, and dinner in the South Beach Diet:

Week 1:

Day 1:
Breakfast: Vegetable Omelet

Lunch: Grilled Chicken Salad

Dinner: Baked Lemon Herb Chicken

Day 2:

Breakfast: Greek Yogurt with Berries

Lunch: Tuna Lettuce Wraps

Dinner: Cauliflower Rice Stir-Fry

Day 3:

Breakfast: Crustless Quiche

Lunch: Eggplant and Mozzarella Stacks

Dinner: Shrimp and Zucchini Noodles

Day 4:

Breakfast: Turkey and Egg Breakfast Casserole

Lunch: Turkey and Avocado Roll-Ups

Dinner: Turkey and Spinach Meatballs

Day 5:

Breakfast: Ricotta and Cinnamon Pancakes

Lunch: Salmon and Asparagus Foil Packs

Dinner: Grilled Steak with Roasted Vegetables

Day 6:

Breakfast: Egg and Vegetable Muffins

Lunch: Cauliflower Rice Sushi Rolls

Dinner: Baked Cod with Lemon and Dill

Day 7:

Breakfast: Smoked Salmon Roll-Ups

Lunch: Mediterranean Tuna Salad

Dinner: Eggplant Lasagna

Week 2:

Day 8:

Breakfast: Avocado and Egg Salad

Lunch: Chicken and Vegetable Skewers

Dinner: Cabbage and Beef Stir-Fry

Day 9:

Breakfast: Cottage Cheese and Almond Bowl

Lunch: Zucchini Noodles with Pesto and Cherry Tomatoes

Dinner: Lemon Garlic Roasted Chicken Thighs

Day 10:

Breakfast: Chia Seed Pudding

Lunch: Turkey and Spinach Stuffed Mushrooms

Dinner: Zucchini Boats with Ground Turkey

Day 11:

Breakfast: Vegetable Omelet

Lunch: Grilled Chicken Salad

Dinner: Baked Lemon Herb Chicken

Day 12:

Breakfast: Greek Yogurt with Berries

Lunch: Tuna Lettuce Wraps

Dinner: Cauliflower Rice Stir-Fry

Day 13:

Breakfast: Crustless Quiche

Lunch: Eggplant and Mozzarella Stacks

Dinner: Shrimp and Zucchini Noodles

Day 14:

Breakfast: Turkey and Egg Breakfast Casserole

Lunch: Turkey and Avocado Roll-Ups

Dinner: Turkey and Spinach Meatballs

This two-week meal plan offers a diverse selection of Phase One recipes for breakfast, lunch, and dinner, ensuring variety while adhering to the South Beach Diet guidelines. Feel free to adjust portions and ingredients as per personal preferences and dietary needs.

Tips for Success During Phase One

Meal Prepping: Plan and prepare meals in advance to avoid impulsive choices.

Stay Hydrated: To prevent hunger, sip water frequently throughout the day.

Portion Control: Pay attention to recommended portion sizes to avoid overeating.

Mindful Eating: Savor every meal, eat carefully, and pay attention to your body's hunger signals.

Avoid Temptations: Remove unhealthy snacks from your surroundings to minimize temptation.

Support System: Seek support from family or friends following similar dietary goals.

Keep a Food Diary: Track meals and snacks to stay accountable and monitor progress.

Be Patient: Understand that the initial phase might be challenging, but results will follow.

Phase Two: Reintroducing Carbs and Sustained Weight Loss

Phase Two Introduction and Guidelines

The South Beach Diet's second phase is a transitional phase that keeps promoting weight loss while reintroducing nutritious carbohydrates. By gradually adding moderate amounts of whole grains, fruits, and extra veggies back into the diet while adhering to the Phase One guidelines, this phase seeks to increase the variety of foods available to the body.

Goal: Reintroduce nutritious carbohydrates gradually in order to maintain weight loss and create a balanced eating schedule.

Duration: You stay in this phase till you attain your target weight.

Important Rules:

Reintroduction of Carbohydrates: Reintroduce fruits, whole grains, and certain starchy vegetables to meals gradually.

Portion Control: To guarantee balanced meals, keep portion sizes consistent.

Balanced Meals: Keep focusing on veggies, lean meats, healthy fats, and now, moderate amounts of whole carbohydrates.

Tracking Progress: Keep a close eye on your weight and evaluate how reintroducing carbohydrates impacts your ability to lose weight.

Phase Two Meal Recipes

Breakfast Recipes

Mediterranean Omelet

Preparation Time: 10 minutes
Cooking Time: 10 minutes
Total Time: 20 minutes
Servings: 2

Ingredients:

- 4 large eggs
- 1/4 cup crumbled feta cheese
- 1/4 cup chopped sun-dried tomatoes
- 1/4 cup chopped Kalamata olives
- 1/4 cup chopped fresh spinach

1/4 teaspoon dried oregano

Salt and pepper to taste

1 tablespoon olive oil

Directions:

➢ In a medium bowl, whisk together the eggs, feta cheese, sun-dried tomatoes, Kalamata olives, spinach, oregano, salt, and pepper.

➢ In a nonstick skillet, warm the olive oil over medium heat.

➢ Once the oil is hot, pour the egg mixture into the skillet and cook until the edges start to set, about 2-3 minutes.

➢ Gently raise the omelet's edges with a spatula to allow the raw eggs to spill out underneath.

➢ Once the top of the omelet is almost set, fold it in half and cook for another 1-2 minutes until the eggs are fully cooked.

➢ Serve the omelet hot with a side of toast or fresh fruit.

Whole Grain Blueberry Pancakes

Preparation Time: 15 minutes

Cooking Time: 10 minutes

Total Time: 25 minutes

Servings: 4

Ingredients:

- 1 cup whole wheat flour
- 2 tablespoons brown sugar
- 2 teaspoons baking powder
- 1/2 teaspoon baking soda
- 1/4 teaspoon salt
- 1 cup buttermilk
- 1 large egg
- 2 tablespoons unsalted butter, melted
- 1 teaspoon vanilla extract
- 1 cup fresh blueberries
- Butter or oil for cooking
- Maple syrup for serving

Directions:

➢ In a large bowl, whisk together the whole wheat flour, brown sugar, baking powder, baking soda, and salt.

- In another bowl, whisk the buttermilk, egg, melted butter, and vanilla extract until well combined.
- After adding the wet components to the dry ingredients, mix just until incorporated. The batter may be slightly lumpy. Be careful not to overmix.
- Gently fold in the fresh blueberries.
- Place a non-stick skillet or griddle over medium heat and add a small amount of butter or oil.
- Once the skillet is hot, pour 1/4 cup of batter for each pancake. Cook until the edges look set and bubbles form on the surface, then flip and cook until golden brown on the other side.
- Continue with the remaining batter, adjusting the skillet's oil or butter content as necessary.
- Serve the pancakes warm with maple syrup.

Avocado and Tomato Breakfast Sandwich

Preparation Time: 10 minutes

Cooking Time: 5 minutes

Total Time: 15 minutes

Servings: 2

Ingredients:

- 4 slices whole grain bread
- 1 ripe avocado, mashed
- 1 medium tomato, sliced
- 2 large eggs
- Salt and pepper to taste
- 1 tablespoon olive oil

Directions:

➢ The bread pieces should be toasted till golden brown.

➢ Spread the mashed avocado on two slices of toast.

➢ Top the avocado with the sliced tomato.

➢ Heat olive oil in a skillet that is nonstick over medium heat.

➢ Pour the eggs into the skillet and cook for two to three minutes, or until the yolks are still runny and the whites are set..

- ➤ Add pepper as well as salt to taste when preparing the eggs.
- ➤ Use a spatula to carefully transfer the eggs onto the tomato slices.
- ➤ Top the eggs with the remaining slices of toast.
- ➤ Serve the breakfast sandwich hot with a side of fresh fruit.

Smoked Salmon Bagel

Preparation Time: 10 minutes

Cooking Time: 0 minutes

Total Time: 10 minutes

Servings: 1

Ingredients:

- 1 whole grain bagel, sliced in half
- 2 tablespoons cream cheese
- 2 ounces smoked salmon
- 1 tablespoon capers
- 1 slice red onion
- 1 slice tomato
- Fresh dill for garnish

Directions:

➢ Toast the bagel slices until lightly crispy.
➢ Spread the cream cheese on both halves of the bagel.
➢ Top one half of the bagel with the smoked salmon.
➢ Sprinkle the capers over the smoked salmon.
➢ Add the slice of red onion and the slice of tomato.
➢ Garnish with fresh dill.
➢ Place the second bagel half on top.
➢ Serve the smoked salmon bagel immediately.

Greek Yogurt Parfait

Preparation Time: 10 minutes

Cooking Time: 0 minutes

Total Time: 10 minutes

Servings: 2

Ingredients:

- 1 cup plain Greek yogurt
- 1/2 cup fresh berries (such as strawberries, blueberries, or raspberries)
- 1/4 cup granola
- 1 tablespoon honey

Directions:

➢ In two small glasses or bowls, layer the Greek yogurt, fresh berries, and granola.

➢ Drizzle the honey over the top of each parfait.

➢ Serve the Greek yogurt parfait immediately.

Whole Grain Breakfast Burrito

Preparation Time: 15 minutes

Cooking Time: 10 minutes

Total Time: 25 minutes

Servings: 2

Ingredients:

- 2 whole grain tortillas
- 4 large eggs
- 1/4 cup shredded cheddar cheese
- 1/4 cup chopped fresh spinach
- 1/4 cup chopped fresh tomatoes
- Salt and pepper to taste
- 1 tablespoon olive oil

Directions:

- ➢ In a medium bowl, whisk together the eggs, cheddar cheese, spinach, tomatoes, salt, and pepper.
- ➢ In a nonstick skillet, warm the olive oil over medium heat.
- ➢ Once the oil is hot, pour the egg mixture into the skillet and cook until the eggs are scrambled and fully cooked, about 5-7 minutes.
- ➢ Use a skillet or a microwave to reheat the tortillas.
- ➢ Spoon the two tortillas with the scrambled eggs.
- ➢ Roll up the tortillas into burritos.
- ➢ Serve the whole grain breakfast burritos hot with a side of fresh fruit.

Quinoa Breakfast Bowl

Preparation Time: 10 minutes

Cooking Time: 15 minutes

Total Time: 25 minutes

Servings: 2

Ingredients:

- 1 cup cooked quinoa
- 1 cup mixed fresh berries (strawberries, blueberries, raspberries)
- 1/4 cup chopped nuts (almonds, walnuts, or pecans)
- 1/4 cup Greek yogurt
- 2 tablespoons honey or maple syrup
- 1 teaspoon chia seeds (optional)

Directions:

➢ Divide the cooked quinoa between two bowls.
➢ Top each bowl of quinoa with mixed fresh berries and chopped nuts.
➢ Add a dollop of Greek yogurt on top of the berries.
➢ Drizzle honey or maple syrup over the bowls.
➢ Sprinkle chia seeds on top if desired.
➢ Serve the quinoa breakfast bowls immediately as a nutritious and filling breakfast option.

Whole Grain French Toast

Preparation Time: 10 minutes

Cooking Time: 10 minutes

Total Time: 20 minutes

Servings: 4

Ingredients:

- 8 slices whole grain bread
- 4 large eggs
- 1/2 cup milk
- 1 teaspoon vanilla extract
- 1 teaspoon ground cinnamon
- 1 tablespoon butter for cooking
- Maple syrup or fruit for topping (optional)

Directions:

- ➢ Combine the eggs, milk, ground cinnamon, and vanilla essence in a shallow basin.
- ➢ Dip each slice of whole grain bread into the egg mixture, ensuring both sides are coated but not soaked.
- ➢ In a pan or griddle above a medium-high flame, melt butter.
- ➢ Cook the bread slices for about 3-4 minutes per side or until they're golden brown and cooked through.
- ➢ Remove the French toast from the skillet and serve warm.
- ➢ Top with maple syrup or your favorite fruit if desired.

Vegetable Frittata

Preparation Time: 10 minutes

Cooking Time: 20 minutes

Total Time: 30 minutes

Servings: 4

Ingredients:

- 8 large eggs
- 1 cup chopped mixed vegetables (bell peppers, onions, spinach, mushrooms, etc.)
- 1/2 cup shredded cheddar cheese
- 2 tablespoons olive oil
- 2 tablespoons milk (optional)
- Salt and pepper to taste

Directions:

➤ Preheat the oven to 350°F (175°C).

➤ In a bowl, whisk together eggs, milk (if using), salt, and pepper until well combined.

➤ In a skillet that is oven-safe, warm the olive oil over medium heat.

➤ Add chopped vegetables to the skillet and sauté until they're slightly tender.

➢ Over the veggies in the skillet, pour the egg whisked mixture.

➢ Cook for 3-4 minutes on the stovetop without stirring until the edges begin to set.

➢ Sprinkle shredded cheddar cheese evenly over the top of the frittata.

➢ Transfer the skillet to the preheated oven and bake for about 12-15 minutes or until the frittata is set and the top is golden.

➢ Take it out of the oven and let it cool down a few minutes before slicing.

➢ Serve the vegetable frittata warm or at room temperature.

Whole Grain Breakfast Wrap

Preparation Time: 10 minutes

Cooking Time: 5 minutes

Total Time: 15 minutes

Servings: 2

Ingredients:

2 large whole grain wraps or tortillas

4 large eggs

1/4 cup chopped bell peppers (any color)

1/4 cup chopped onions

1/4 cup shredded cheese (cheddar, mozzarella, or your choice)

1 avocado, sliced

Salsa or hot sauce for serving (optional)

Salt and pepper to taste

Olive oil for cooking

Directions:

➤ Stir the eggs and add salt and pepper to taste in a bowl.

➤ Heating the olive oil in a big skillet over medium heat.

➤ Add chopped bell peppers and onions to the skillet and sauté until they're softened.

➤ Pour the beaten eggs into the skillet with the peppers and onions.

- ➢ Scramble the eggs until cooked through.
- ➢ Warm the whole grain wraps or tortillas in the microwave or a separate skillet.
- ➢ Place the cooked eggs in the center of each wrap.
- ➢ Top with shredded cheese and avocado slices.
- ➢ Add salsa or hot sauce if desired.
- ➢ Fold in the sides of the wraps and roll them up tightly into breakfast wraps.
- ➢ Serve the whole grain breakfast wraps immediately.
- ➢ These detailed recipes for breakfast dishes, including burritos, bowls, toasts, and wraps, offer variety and wholesome options for your morning meals.

Lunch Recipes

Mediterranean Chicken Salad

Preparation Time: 20 minutes

Total Time: 20 minutes

Servings: 4

Ingredients:

- Two cups of cooked, chopped or shredded chicken breast
- 4 cups mixed salad greens
- 1 cup cherry tomatoes, halved

- 1 cucumber, sliced

- 1/2 red onion, thinly sliced

- 1/2 cup Kalamata olives, pitted

- 1/2 cup crumbled feta cheese

- 1/4 cup chopped fresh parsley

For the Dressing:

1/4 cup extra-virgin olive oil

2 tablespoons red wine vinegar

1 clove garlic, minced

1 teaspoon dried oregano

Salt and pepper to taste

Directions:

- ➢ In a large salad bowl, combine the mixed greens, cherry tomatoes, cucumber slices, red onion, Kalamata olives, and cooked chicken.
- ➢ In a separate small bowl, whisk together the olive oil, red wine vinegar, minced garlic, dried oregano, salt, and pepper to prepare the dressing.
- ➢ After adding the dressing to the salad, gently toss to coat everything equally.
- ➢ Sprinkle crumbled feta cheese and chopped fresh parsley over the salad as a final touch.
- ➢ Serve the Mediterranean chicken salad immediately as a satisfying and flavorful meal.

Whole Grain Veggie Wrap

Preparation Time: 15 minutes

Total Time: 15 minutes

Servings: 2

Ingredients:

- 2 large whole grain wraps or tortillas
- 1 cup hummus
- 1 cup mixed salad greens
- 1 bell pepper, thinly sliced
- 1/2 cucumber, julienned
- 1 carrot, julienned
- 1/2 red onion, thinly sliced
- 1/2 cup crumbled feta cheese (optional)
- Salt and pepper to taste

Directions:

- ➢ Lay out the whole grain wraps or tortillas on a clean surface.
- ➢ Spread a generous amount of hummus over each wrap, leaving a small border around the edges.
- ➢ Layer mixed salad greens, bell pepper slices, julienned cucumber, julienned carrot, and thinly sliced red onion on each wrap.

- ➤ If using, sprinkle crumbled feta cheese evenly over the vegetables.
- ➤ Season with salt and pepper to taste.
- ➤ Roll up the wraps tightly, folding in the sides as you go to secure the fillings.
- ➤ Cut each wrap in half diagonally and serve the whole grain veggie wraps immediately or wrap them tightly in foil for later.

Quinoa and Black Bean Bowl

Preparation Time: 15 minutes

Cooking Time: 15 minutes

Total Time: 30 minutes

Servings: 4

Ingredients:

- 1 cup quinoa, rinsed
- 2 cups water or vegetable broth
- A single can (15 oz) of black beans, washed and drained
- 1 cup corn kernels (fresh, frozen, or canned)
- 1 red bell pepper, diced
- 1/4 cup chopped fresh cilantro
- 2 tablespoons lime juice
- 2 tablespoons olive oil
- 1 teaspoon ground cumin
- Salt and pepper to taste
- Avocado slices for garnish (optional)

Directions:

➢ Quinoa should be combined with water or vegetable broth in a saucepan. Bring to a boil, then reduce heat to low, cover, and simmer for 15 minutes or until the liquid is absorbed and quinoa is cooked.

- ➢ In a large mixing bowl, combine cooked quinoa, black beans, corn kernels, diced red bell pepper, and chopped cilantro.
- ➢ To make the dressing, combine the lime juice, olive oil, ground cumin, salt, and pepper in a small bowl.
- ➢ Pour the dressing over the quinoa and black bean mixture. Toss gently to coat everything evenly.
- ➢ Adjust seasoning if needed.
- ➢ Serve the quinoa and black bean bowl in individual bowls, garnished with avocado slices if desired.

Whole Grain Tuna Salad Sandwich

Preparation Time: 10 minutes

Total Time: 10 minutes

Servings: 2

Ingredients:

- 1 can (5 oz) tuna, drained
- 1/4 cup Greek yogurt
- 2 tablespoons mayonnaise
- 1 celery stalk, finely chopped
- 1 tablespoon red onion, finely chopped
- 1 tablespoon chopped fresh parsley
- 1 teaspoon Dijon mustard
- Salt and pepper to taste
- 4 slices whole grain bread
- Lettuce leaves
- Tomato slices

Directions:

➢ In a mixing bowl, combine drained tuna, Greek yogurt, mayonnaise, chopped celery, chopped red onion, chopped parsley, Dijon mustard, salt, and pepper. Mix until well combined.

- ➢ Lay out the whole grain bread slices on a clean surface.
- ➢ Place lettuce leaves on two bread slices.
- ➢ Top the lettuce leaves with the prepared tuna salad mixture.
- ➢ Add tomato slices on top of the tuna salad.
- ➢ Place the remaining bread slices on top to form sandwiches.
- ➢ Cut each sandwich in half diagonally and serve the whole grain tuna salad sandwiches immediately.

Mediterranean Veggie Pita

Preparation Time: 15 minutes

Total Time: 15 minutes

Servings: 2

Ingredients:

- 2 whole grain pitas, cut in half
- 1 cup hummus
- 1 cup mixed salad greens
- 1/2 cup cherry tomatoes, halved
- 1/2 cucumber, sliced
- 1/4 red onion, thinly sliced
- 1/4 cup Kalamata olives, pitted and sliced
- 2 tablespoons crumbled feta cheese
- Fresh parsley for garnish (optional)
- Olive oil for drizzling (optional)
- Salt and pepper to taste

Directions:

- ➤ Open each half of the whole grain pitas to create pockets.
- ➤ Spread a generous amount of hummus inside each pita pocket.

- ➤ Stuff each pita pocket with mixed salad greens, cherry tomato halves, cucumber slices, thinly sliced red onion, Kalamata olive slices, and crumbled feta cheese.
- ➤ Season with salt and pepper to taste.
- ➤ Garnish with fresh parsley and drizzle with olive oil if desired.
- ➤ Serve the Mediterranean veggie pitas immediately.

Whole Grain Turkey and Avocado Wrap

Preparation Time: 15 minutes

Total Time: 15 minutes

Servings: 2

Ingredients:

- 2 large whole grain wraps or tortillas
- 1 cup cooked turkey breast, sliced
- 1 avocado, sliced
- 1 cup mixed salad greens
- 1/2 cup shredded carrots
- 1/4 cup sliced red bell pepper
- 1/4 cup sliced red onion
- 2 tablespoons Greek yogurt or mayo (optional)
- Salt and pepper to taste

Directions:

➢ Lay out the whole grain wraps or tortillas on a clean surface.

➢ If desired, spread a thin layer of Greek yogurt or mayo on each wrap.

➤ Layer sliced turkey breast, avocado slices, mixed salad greens, shredded carrots, sliced red bell pepper, and sliced red onion on each wrap.

➤ Season with salt and pepper to taste.

➤ Roll up the wraps tightly, folding in the sides as you go to secure the fillings.

➤ Cut each wrap in half diagonally and serve the whole grain turkey and avocado wraps immediately.

Quinoa and Chickpea Salad

Preparation Time: 15 minutes

Cooking Time: 15 minutes

Total Time: 30 minutes

Servings: 4

Ingredients:

- 1 cup quinoa, rinsed
- 2 cups water or vegetable broth
- Quinoa, rinsed and drained, in one can (15 oz).
- 1 cup cherry tomatoes, halved
- 1 cucumber, diced
- 1/2 red onion, finely chopped
- 1/4 cup chopped fresh parsley
- 2 tablespoons olive oil
- 2 tablespoons lemon juice
- 1 teaspoon ground cumin
- Salt and pepper to taste

Directions:

➢ Quinoa should be combined with water or vegetable broth in a saucepan. Bring to a boil, then reduce heat to low, cover, and simmer for 15 minutes or until the liquid is absorbed and quinoa is cooked.

- ➤ In a large mixing bowl, combine cooked quinoa, drained and rinsed chickpeas, cherry tomatoes, diced cucumber, finely chopped red onion, and chopped fresh parsley.
- ➤ In a small bowl, whisk together olive oil, lemon juice, ground cumin, salt, and pepper to create the dressing.
- ➤ Over the quinoa & chickpea mixture, drizzle the dressing. Toss gently to coat everything evenly.
- ➤ Adjust seasoning if needed.
- ➤ Serve the quinoa and chickpea salad in individual bowls as a wholesome and satisfying meal.

Whole Grain Caprese Panini

Preparation Time: 10 minutes

Cooking Time: 5 minutes

Total Time: 15 minutes

Servings: 2

Ingredients:

- 4 slices whole grain bread
- 4 slices mozzarella cheese
- 1 large tomato, thinly sliced
- 1/4 cup fresh basil leaves
- 2 tablespoons balsamic glaze (optional)
- Olive oil or butter for cooking

Directions:

➢ Preheat a skillet, grill pan, or panini press over medium heat.

➢ Lay out the whole grain bread slices on a clean surface.

➢ Place a slice of mozzarella cheese on two bread slices.

➢ Top the cheese with thinly sliced tomatoes and fresh basil leaves.

➢ Drizzle balsamic glaze over the basil leaves if desired.

➢ Place the remaining bread slices on top to form sandwiches.

- ➤ Brush the outer sides of each sandwich with olive oil or spread butter.
- ➤ Place the sandwiches in the heated panini press, grill pan, or skillet.
- ➤ Cook for about 2-3 minutes on each side until the bread is golden brown and the cheese is melted.
- ➤ Remove from the heat, slice the sandwiches in half diagonally, and serve the whole grain Caprese panini immediately.

Mediterranean Hummus Plate

Preparation Time: 10 minutes

Total Time: 10 minutes

Servings: 2

Ingredients:

- 1 cup hummus
- 1/2 cup cherry tomatoes, halved
- 1/2 cucumber, sliced
- 1/4 red onion, thinly sliced
- 1/4 cup Kalamata olives, pitted
- 2 tablespoons crumbled feta cheese
- 2 tablespoons chopped fresh parsley
- Whole grain pita bread or pita chips for serving

Directions:

➢ Spread a generous amount of hummus on a serving plate.

➢ Arrange cherry tomatoes, cucumber slices, thinly sliced red onion, Kalamata olives, crumbled feta cheese, and chopped fresh parsley on top of the hummus.

➢ Serve the Mediterranean hummus plate with whole grain pita bread or pita chips for dipping.

Whole Grain Veggie Burger

Preparation Time: 20 minutes

Cooking Time: 10 minutes

Total Time: 30 minutes

Servings: 4

Ingredients:

- 4 whole grain burger buns
- 4 whole grain veggie burger patties (store-bought or homemade)
- 1 cup mixed salad greens
- 1 large tomato, sliced
- 1 avocado, sliced
- 1/4 red onion, thinly sliced
- 4 tablespoons hummus or Greek yogurt sauce (optional)
- Olive oil for cooking

Directions:

➢ If using store-bought veggie burger patties, follow the package instructions to cook them.

➢ If making homemade veggie patties, cook them in a skillet with a little olive oil over medium heat for about 4-5 minutes per side or until heated through and golden brown.

- ➢ Halve all of the grain burger buns and give them a quick toast.
- ➢ Spread hummus or Greek yogurt sauce on the bottom halves of the buns if desired.
- ➢ Place a cooked veggie burger patty on each bottom bun.
- ➢ Top the patties with mixed salad greens, tomato slices, avocado slices, and thinly sliced red onion.
- ➢ Place the top half of the buns on top.
- ➢ Serve the whole grain veggie burgers immediately.

These recipes offer a wide array of delicious, nutritious, and satisfying options using whole grains, vegetables, and various ingredients.

Dinner Recipes

Whole Grain Spaghetti with Turkey Meatballs

Preparation Time: 20 minutes

Cooking Time: 30 minutes

Total Time: 50 minutes

Servings: 4

Ingredients:

For the Meatballs:

- 1 pound ground turkey
- 1/2 cup whole grain breadcrumbs
- 1/4 cup grated Parmesan cheese
- 1 large egg
- 2 cloves garlic, minced
- 2 tablespoons chopped fresh parsley
- 1 teaspoon dried oregano
- Salt and pepper to taste
- 2 tablespoons olive oil

For the Pasta:

- 8 ounces whole grain spaghetti
- 2 cups marinara sauce (store-bought or homemade)

➢ Fresh basil leaves for garnish (optional)

Directions:

➢ Preheat the oven to 400°F (200°C).

➢ In a mixing bowl, combine ground turkey, whole grain breadcrumbs, grated Parmesan cheese, egg, minced garlic, chopped fresh parsley, dried oregano, salt, and pepper. Mix until well combined.

➢ Form the ingredients into meatballs with a diameter of about one inch.

➢ In a skillet that is oven-safe, warm the olive oil over medium heat.

➢ Brown the meatballs on all sides in the skillet, about 2-3 minutes per side.

➢ Transfer the skillet to the preheated oven and bake for 10-12 minutes or until the meatballs are cooked through.

➢ Meanwhile, cook whole grain spaghetti according to package instructions until al dente.

➢ Heat marinara sauce in a separate saucepan.

➢ When the meatballs are done, remove them from the oven.

➢ Serve the whole grain spaghetti topped with marinara sauce and turkey meatballs. If desired, garnish with freshly picked basil leaves.

Mediterranean Baked Cod

Preparation Time: 15 minutes

Cooking Time: 20 minutes

Total Time: 35 minutes

Servings: 4

Ingredients:

- 4 cod fillets (6 ounces each)
- 1/4 cup olive oil
- 2 cloves garlic, minced
- 2 tablespoons lemon juice
- 1 teaspoon dried oregano
- 1 teaspoon paprika
- Salt and pepper to taste
- Lemon wedges for serving
- Chopped fresh parsley for garnish

Directions:

➢ Preheat the oven to 400°F (200°C). Lightly coat a baking dish with olive oil.

➢ Place cod fillets in the prepared baking dish.

- ➢ In a small bowl, whisk together olive oil, minced garlic, lemon juice, dried oregano, paprika, salt, and pepper to create the marinade.
- ➢ Pour the marinade over the cod fillets, ensuring they are evenly coated.
- ➢ Bake the fish for 15 to 20 minutes in a preheated oven, or until it is opaque and flake easily with a fork.
- ➢ Remove the baked cod from the oven and garnish with chopped fresh parsley.
- ➢ Serve the Mediterranean baked cod with lemon wedges on the side.

Whole Grain Pesto Shrimp Pasta

Preparation Time: 15 minutes

Cooking Time: 15 minutes

Total Time: 30 minutes

Servings: 4

Ingredients:

- 8 ounces whole grain pasta
- 1 pound large shrimp, peeled and deveined
- 3 tablespoons pesto sauce (store-bought or homemade)
- 2 tablespoons olive oil
- 3 cloves garlic, minced
- 1 cup cherry tomatoes, halved
- Salt and pepper to taste
- Fresh basil leaves for garnish (optional)
- Grated Parmesan cheese for serving (optional)

Directions:

- ➤ Cook whole grain pasta according to package instructions until al dente. Drain and set aside.
- ➤ In a skillet, heat olive oil over medium-high heat.
- ➤ Garlic powder should be added to the skillet and cooked for 30 seconds or less, or until aromatic.

- ➤ Add shrimp to the skillet and cook for 2-3 minutes per side until they turn pink and opaque.
- ➤ Stir in pesto sauce and halved cherry tomatoes. Cook for an additional 1-2 minutes.
- ➤ Add the cooked whole grain pasta to the skillet with the shrimp and toss to coat evenly.
- ➤ Season with salt and pepper to taste.
- ➤ Garnish with fresh basil leaves and serve the whole grain pesto shrimp pasta. If preferred, top with grated Parmesan cheese.

Mediterranean Grilled Veggie Platter

Preparation Time: 20 minutes

Cooking Time: 10 minutes

Total Time: 30 minutes

Servings: 4

Ingredients:

- 2 zucchinis, sliced lengthwise
- 2 yellow squash, sliced lengthwise
- 1 eggplant, sliced
- 2 bell peppers (assorted colors), halved and seeded
- 1 red onion, sliced into thick rounds
- 1/4 cup olive oil
- 3 cloves garlic, minced
- 2 tablespoons balsamic vinegar
- 1 teaspoon dried oregano
- Salt and pepper to taste
- Fresh parsley for garnish

Directions:

➢ Turn the heat up to medium-high on a grill or grill pan.

- In a bowl, combine olive oil, minced garlic, balsamic vinegar, dried oregano, salt, and pepper to create the marinade.
- Brush both sides of the sliced vegetables with the marinade.
- Place the vegetables on the grill and cook for 3-4 minutes per side or until they have grill marks and are tender.
- Arrange the grilled vegetables on a platter.
- Drizzle any remaining marinade over the vegetables.
- Garnish with fresh parsley and serve the Mediterranean grilled veggie platter as a delightful side dish.

Whole Grain Chicken and Broccoli Stir-Fry

Preparation Time: 15 minutes

Cooking Time: 15 minutes

Total Time: 30 minutes

Servings: 4

Ingredients:

- 1 pound boneless, skinless chicken breasts, thinly sliced
- 2 cups broccoli florets
- 1 red bell pepper, sliced
- 1 yellow bell pepper, sliced
- 3 cloves garlic, minced
- 2 tablespoons soy sauce
- 2 tablespoons oyster sauce
- 1 tablespoon honey
- 2 tablespoons olive oil
- 2 tablespoons water or chicken broth
- Sesame seeds for garnish (optional)
- Cooked whole grain rice for serving

Directions:

- In a small bowl, whisk together soy sauce, oyster sauce, honey, and water or chicken broth to create the sauce.
- In a big skillet or wok, heat the olive oil over a medium-high temperature.
- Add the minced garlic and cook it for a few seconds, until it becomes aromatic.
- Add sliced chicken to the skillet and stir-fry for 3-4 minutes until it's no longer pink.
- Add broccoli florets and sliced bell peppers to the skillet. Continue stir-frying for an additional 3-4 minutes until the vegetables are tender-crisp and the chicken is cooked through.
- Pour the prepared sauce into the skillet and toss everything together until the chicken and vegetables are evenly coated.
- Cook for another 1-2 minutes, allowing the sauce to thicken slightly.
- Remove from heat and sprinkle sesame seeds over the stir-fry if desired.
- Serve the whole grain chicken and broccoli stir-fry immediately over cooked whole grain rice.

Mediterranean Stuffed Bell Peppers

Preparation Time: 20 minutes

Cooking Time: 40 minutes

Total Time: 1 hour

Servings: 4

Ingredients:

- 4 large bell peppers (any color), halved and seeds removed
- 1 cup cooked quinoa
- One can (15 oz) of cleaned and drained chickpeas
- 1 cup cherry tomatoes, halved
- 1/2 cup chopped fresh spinach
- 1/4 cup chopped fresh parsley
- 1/4 cup crumbled feta cheese
- 2 tablespoons olive oil
- 2 cloves garlic, minced
- 1 teaspoon dried oregano
- Salt and pepper to taste

Directions:

➢ Preheat the oven to 375°F (190°C). Grease a baking dish lightly.

- ➢ Place the bell pepper halves in the prepared baking dish, cut-side up.
- ➢ In a mixing bowl, combine cooked quinoa, drained and rinsed chickpeas, cherry tomatoes, chopped fresh spinach, chopped fresh parsley, crumbled feta cheese, minced garlic, dried oregano, salt, and pepper.
- ➢ Drizzle olive oil over the quinoa mixture and toss to combine.
- ➢ Spoon the quinoa mixture into each bell pepper half, pressing gently to fill them.
- ➢ Cover the baking dish with foil and bake for 25-30 minutes.
- ➢ Remove the foil and bake for an additional 10-15 minutes until the bell peppers are tender and the filling is heated through.
- ➢ Serve the Mediterranean stuffed bell peppers warm.

Whole Grain Teriyaki Salmon

Preparation Time: 15 minutes

Cooking Time: 15 minutes

Total Time: 30 minutes

Servings: 4

Ingredients:

- 4 salmon fillets (6 ounces each), skin-on
- 1/4 cup low-sodium soy sauce
- 2 tablespoons honey
- 2 tablespoons rice vinegar
- 1 tablespoon sesame oil
- 2 cloves garlic, minced
- 1 teaspoon grated fresh ginger
- 2 tablespoons chopped green onions (for garnish, optional)
- Sesame seeds (for garnish, optional)
- Cooked whole grain rice or quinoa for serving

Directions:

➤ Preheat the oven to 400°F (200°C). Grease a baking sheet gently or line it with parchment paper.

➢ In a bowl, mix together soy sauce, honey, rice vinegar, sesame oil, minced garlic, and grated ginger to create the teriyaki sauce.

➢ Skin-side down, put the salmon fillets on the sheet of baking parchment that has been prepared.

➢ Pour half of the teriyaki sauce over the salmon fillets, ensuring they are coated evenly.

➢ Bake for 12 to 15 minutes, or until a fork can easily pierce the salmon, in a preheated oven.

➢ While the salmon is baking, pour the remaining teriyaki sauce into a small saucepan.

➢ Simmer the sauce over medium heat for 3-5 minutes until it thickens slightly.

➢ Once the salmon is done, remove it from the oven and drizzle with the thickened teriyaki sauce.

➢ Sprinkle chopped green onions and sesame seeds over the salmon if desired.

➢ Serve the whole grain teriyaki salmon alongside cooked whole grain rice or quinoa.

Mediterranean Lentil Soup

Preparation Time: 15 minutes

Cooking Time: 45 minutes

Total Time: 1 hour

Servings: 6

Ingredients:

- 1 cup dry brown lentils, rinsed
- 1 onion, finely chopped
- 2 carrots, diced
- 2 celery stalks, diced
- 3 cloves garlic, minced
- 6 cups low-sodium vegetable or chicken broth
- 1 can (14 oz) diced tomatoes
- 2 tablespoons tomato paste
- 1 teaspoon dried thyme
- 1 teaspoon ground cumin
- 1 bay leaf
- Salt and pepper to taste
- Fresh parsley for garnish (optional)
- Lemon wedges for serving (optional)

Directions:

- ➤ Heat olive oil in a big pot or Dutch oven over medium heat.
- ➤ Add chopped onions, diced carrots, and diced celery. They should start to soften after about five minutes of sautéing.
- ➤ Cook the minced garlic for one to two more minutes after adding it.
- ➤ Stir in rinsed brown lentils, vegetable or chicken broth, diced tomatoes, tomato paste, dried thyme, ground cumin, bay leaf, salt, and pepper.
- ➤ Bring the soup to a boil, then reduce heat to low, cover, and simmer for 30-40 minutes or until the lentils are tender.
- ➤ Remove the bay leaf from the soup.
- ➤ Use an immersion blender or transfer a portion of the soup to a blender and blend until you reach your desired consistency.
- ➤ Serve the Mediterranean lentil soup garnished with fresh parsley and accompanied by lemon wedges if desired.

Whole Grain Turkey and Black Bean Tacos

Preparation Time: 15 minutes

Cooking Time: 15 minutes

Total Time: 30 minutes

Servings: 4

Ingredients:

- 1 tablespoon olive oil
- 1 pound ground turkey
- 1 packet (1.25 oz) taco seasoning mix
- One can (15 oz) of cleaned and rinsed black beans
- 1 cup corn kernels (fresh, frozen, or canned)
- 1/2 cup salsa
- 8 whole grain taco shells or tortillas
- Toppings: shredded lettuce, diced tomatoes, diced avocado, shredded cheese, chopped cilantro, lime wedges, sour cream (optional)

Directions:

- ➢ Heat olive oil in a pan over a medium-high heat.
- ➢ Add ground turkey to the skillet and cook, breaking it up with a spoon, until it's browned and cooked through.

- As directed on the package, stir in the seasoning for tacos mix.
- Add black beans and corn kernels to the skillet. Cook for a further three to four minutes, or until well heated.
- Warm the whole grain taco shells or tortillas according to package instructions.
- Spoon the turkey and black bean mixture into the taco shells or tortillas.
- Top with shredded lettuce, diced tomatoes, diced avocado, shredded cheese, chopped cilantro, and a squeeze of lime juice if desired.
- Serve the whole grain turkey and black bean tacos immediately with optional toppings.

These recipes offer a diverse range of flavorful and wholesome dishes using whole grains, lean proteins, and a variety of vegetables.

Phase Two Meal Plan Structure

Here's a two-week meal plan structure incorporating the provided Phase Two recipes for breakfast, lunch, and dinner in the South Beach Diet:

Week 1

Day 1:

Breakfast: Mediterranean Omelet

Lunch: Mediterranean Chicken Salad

Dinner: Whole Grain Spaghetti with Turkey Meatballs

Day 2:

Breakfast: Whole Grain Blueberry Pancakes

Lunch: Whole Grain Veggie Wrap

Dinner: Mediterranean Baked Cod

Day 3:

Breakfast: Avocado and Tomato Breakfast Sandwich

Lunch: Quinoa and Black Bean Bowl

Dinner: Whole Grain Pesto Shrimp Pasta

Day 4:

Breakfast: Smoked Salmon Bagel

Lunch: Whole Grain Tuna Salad Sandwich

Dinner: Mediterranean Grilled Veggie Platter

Day 5:

Breakfast: Greek Yogurt Parfait

Lunch: Mediterranean Veggie Pita

Dinner: Whole Grain Chicken and Broccoli Stir-Fry

Day 6:

Breakfast: Whole Grain Breakfast Burrito

Lunch: Whole Grain Turkey and Avocado Wrap

Dinner: Mediterranean Stuffed Bell Peppers

Day 7:

Breakfast: Quinoa Breakfast Bowl

Lunch: Quinoa and Chickpea Salad

Dinner: Whole Grain Teriyaki Salmon

Week 2

Day 8:

Breakfast: Whole Grain French Toast

Lunch: Whole Grain Caprese Panini

Dinner: Mediterranean Lentil Soup

Day 9:

Breakfast: Vegetable Frittata

Lunch: Mediterranean Hummus Plate

Dinner: Whole Grain Turkey and Black Bean Tacos

Day 10:

Breakfast: Whole Grain Breakfast Wrap

Lunch: Whole Grain Veggie Burger

Dinner: Mediterranean Baked Cod

Day 11:

Breakfast: Mediterranean Omelet

Lunch: Mediterranean Chicken Salad

Dinner: Whole Grain Spaghetti with Turkey Meatballs

Day 12:

Breakfast: Whole Grain Blueberry Pancakes

Lunch: Whole Grain Veggie Wrap

Dinner: Mediterranean Grilled Veggie Platter

Day 13:

Breakfast: Avocado and Tomato Breakfast Sandwich

Lunch: Quinoa and Black Bean Bowl

Dinner: Whole Grain Pesto Shrimp Pasta

Day 14:

Breakfast: Smoked Salmon Bagel

Lunch: Whole Grain Tuna Salad Sandwich

Dinner: Mediterranean Stuffed Bell Peppers

This two-week meal plan provides a variety of Phase Two recipes for breakfast, lunch, and dinner, offering diverse flavors and nutrient-rich meals while incorporating healthy whole grains, lean proteins, and vegetables as per the South Beach Diet guidelines. Adjust portions and ingredients based on personal preferences and dietary needs.

Phase Three: Maintenance and Healthy Lifestyle

Phase Three Overview and Guidelines

Phase Three of the South Beach Diet is a sustainable way of living that emphasizes preserving weight loss, enhancing general health, and creating enduring habits. It integrates the concepts acquired in Phases One and Two into a lifetime dietary pattern, emphasizing a balanced approach to eating.

Goals: To keep a healthy weight, maintain good habits, and guarantee long-term health.

Duration: The adoption of a lifetime, healthy eating routine is symbolized by this ongoing phase.

Important Rules:

Maintain a balanced diet by giving lean proteins, healthy fats, whole grains, fruits, and vegetables first priority.

Portion Control: To avoid overindulging, be mindful of portion proportions.

Eat mindfully by being aware of your body's signals of hunger and fullness.

Frequent Exercise: For general health and well-being, make time for physical activity each day.

Flexibility: Permit sporadic excesses while keeping the overall composition of your diet in check.

Phase Three Recipes
Breakfast Recipes

Greek Yogurt with Berries and Almonds

Preparation Time: 5 minutes

Total Time: 5 minutes

Servings: 1

Ingredients:

- 1 cup Greek yogurt
- 1/2 cup mixed berries (blueberries, strawberries, raspberries)
- 2 tablespoons sliced almonds
- Honey or agave nectar (optional, for sweetening)

Directions:

- ➢ Pour Greek yogurt in a serving bowl or plate.
- ➢ Rinse the mixed berries and pat them dry with a paper towel.
- ➢ Top the Greek yogurt with mixed berries and sprinkle sliced almonds over the berries.
- ➢ Drizzle a small amount of honey or agave nectar over the yogurt and berries if desired.
- ➢ Serve immediately and enjoy this nutritious and delicious Greek yogurt with berries and almonds!

Note: Feel free to adjust the quantity of berries and almonds to suit your taste.

Spinach and Feta Omelet

Preparation Time: 10 minutes

Cooking Time: 5 minutes

Total Time: 15 minutes

Servings: 1

Ingredients:

- 2 large eggs
- 1 cup fresh spinach leaves
- 1/4 cup crumbled feta cheese
- 1 tablespoon olive oil or butter
- Salt and pepper to taste

Directions:

➢ Crack the eggs into a bowl, add a pinch of salt and pepper, and beat them lightly with a fork.

➢ In a nonstick skillet, preheat the butter or olive oil over medium heat.

➢ Add fresh spinach leaves to the skillet and sauté for 1-2 minutes until wilted.

➢ Pour the beaten eggs into the skillet over the spinach.

- ➢ Allow the eggs to cook for about 1-2 minutes, gently lifting the edges with a spatula to let the uncooked eggs flow to the bottom.
- ➢ Evenly top one side of the omelet with crumbled feta cheese.
- ➢ Gently fold the remaining omelet half over the side with the cheese.
- ➢ Cook for an additional 1-2 minutes until the cheese melts and the omelet is cooked through.
- ➢ Transfer the omelet to a platter and enjoy it warm.

Avocado and Tomato Breakfast Sandwich

Preparation Time: 10 minutes

Cooking Time: 5 minutes

Total Time: 15 minutes

Servings: 1

Ingredients:

- 2 slices of whole grain bread
- 1 ripe avocado
- 1 tomato, sliced
- 1-2 slices of cheese (optional)
- Salt and pepper to taste

Directions:

➢ Toast the whole grain bread slices to your preferred level of crispiness.

➢ While the bread is toasting, halve the avocado, remove the pit, and scoop out the flesh into a bowl. Mash it with a fork and season with salt and pepper.

➢ On one side of every slice of toasted bread, spread the mashed avocado.

- Layer the tomato slices on top of the mashed avocado on one slice of bread.

- If using cheese, place the cheese slices on top of the tomato slices.

- Top with the other slice of bread, avocado side down, to make a sandwich.

- Optionally, warm the sandwich in a skillet for a minute on each side to melt the cheese and heat through the sandwich.

- Cut the sandwich in half diagonally and serve immediately.

Quinoa Breakfast Bowl

Preparation Time: 10 minutes

Cooking Time: 15 minutes (for quinoa)

Total Time: 25 minutes

Servings: 2

Ingredients:

- 1 cup cooked quinoa
- 1 cup mixed berries (blueberries, strawberries, raspberries)
- 1/4 cup chopped nuts (almonds, walnuts, or pecans)
- 2 tablespoons honey or maple syrup
- 1/2 cup Greek yogurt
- Optional: sliced bananas or other favorite fruits

Directions:

- Prepare quinoa according to package instructions (usually a 1:2 ratio of quinoa to water, simmered for 15 minutes).
- Divide the cooked quinoa between two bowls.
- Top each bowl of quinoa with mixed berries, chopped nuts, and sliced bananas or other favorite fruits if desired.
- Drizzle honey or maple syrup over the bowls for sweetness.
- Add a dollop of Greek yogurt to each bowl.
- Serve immediately and mix the ingredients together when ready to eat.

Whole Grain French Toast

Preparation Time: 10 minutes

Cooking Time: 10 minutes

Total Time: 20 minutes

Servings: 2

Ingredients:

- 4 slices of whole grain bread
- 2 large eggs
- 1/4 cup milk (or almond milk)
- 1 teaspoon vanilla extract
- 1/2 teaspoon ground cinnamon
- Some butter(margarine) or cooking spray (for greasing the pan)
- Optional toppings: Fresh berries, sliced bananas, maple syrup

Directions:

➤ In a shallow dish, whisk together eggs, milk, vanilla extract, and ground cinnamon until well combined.

➤ Dip each slice of whole grain bread into the egg mixture, allowing both sides to absorb the mixture but not become soggy.

- ➤ Grease a non-stick pan or griddle with a cooking spray or margarine and heat it over medium heat.
- ➤ Place the coated bread slices onto the skillet or griddle and cook for about 2-3 minutes on each side, or until golden brown.
- ➤ Once cooked, transfer the French toast slices to a plate.
- ➤ Serve warm and top with fresh berries, sliced bananas, or a drizzle of maple syrup if desired.

Turkey Sausage & Veggie Frittata

Preparation Time: 15 minutes

Cooking Time: 20 minutes

Total Time: 35 minutes

Servings: 4

Ingredients:

- 8 large eggs
- 1/2 cup diced turkey sausage (cooked)
- 1/2 cup diced bell peppers (any color)
- 1/2 cup diced onions
- 1/2 cup chopped spinach or kale
- 1/2 cup shredded cheese (cheddar or mozzarella)
- 1 tablespoon olive oil
- Salt and pepper to taste

Directions:

- ➤ Preheat the oven to 350°F (175°C).
- ➤ In a mixing bowl, whisk together eggs, salt, and pepper until well combined.
- ➤ In a skillet that is oven-safe, warm the olive oil over medium heat.

➢ Add diced onions and bell peppers to the skillet and sauté until softened, about 3-4 minutes.

➢ Add diced turkey sausage and chopped spinach or kale to the skillet, and cook for an additional 2 minutes.

➢ Pour the whisked eggs into the skillet over the sausage and vegetables.

➢ Evenly distribute shredded cheese on top of the frittata.

➢ Once the oven is hot, place the skillet inside and bake for 15 to 20 minutes, up to when the frittata is set in the middle.

➢ Remove from the oven, let it cool slightly, then slice and serve.

Coconut Milk Chia Pudding with Berries

Preparation Time: 5 minutes (plus chilling time)

Total Time: 4 hours (chilling time)

Servings: 2

Ingredients:

- 1/4 cup chia seeds
- 1 cup coconut milk
- 1 tablespoon maple syrup or honey
- 1/2 teaspoon vanilla extract
- 1/2 cup mixed berries (blueberries, raspberries, strawberries)
- Optional toppings: Shredded coconut, sliced almonds

Directions:

➤ In a bowl, mix together chia seeds, coconut milk, maple syrup (or honey), and vanilla extract.

➤ Make sure the chia seeds are dispersed evenly by giving it a good stir.

➤ To help the chia seeds absorb the liquid and become pudding-like, cover the bowl and chill for at least four hours or overnight.

- ➢ Before serving, stir the chia pudding to ensure it's well combined and smooth.
- ➢ Transfer the chia pudding into glasses or bowls for serving.
- ➢ Top the pudding with mixed berries, shredded coconut, sliced almonds, or your desired toppings.
- ➢ Serve chilled and enjoy this creamy coconut milk chia pudding with a burst of fresh berries!

Smoked Salmon & Avocado Scramble

Preparation Time: 10 minutes

Cooking Time: 5 minutes

Total Time: 15 minutes

Servings: 2

Ingredients:

- 4 large eggs
- 4 oz smoked salmon, chopped
- 1 ripe avocado, diced
- 2 tablespoons chopped fresh dill (optional)
- 1 tablespoon butter or olive oil
- Salt and pepper to taste
- Optional: Sliced whole grain toast

Directions:

➤ Crack the eggs into a bowl, add a pinch of salt and pepper, and whisk them until well combined.

➤ Use a skillet over a medium-low flame to melt butter or olive oil.

➤ Add the beaten eggs to the skillet and cook, stirring gently, until they start to set but are still slightly runny.

- ➢ Add chopped smoked salmon to the eggs and continue cooking for another minute, stirring occasionally.
- ➢ Gently fold in diced avocado and chopped fresh dill (if using) into the egg mixture.
- ➢ Cook for an additional 1-2 minutes until the eggs are fully cooked and the avocado is warmed through.
- ➢ Divide the smoked salmon and avocado scramble onto plates.
- ➢ Serve immediately, optionally with slices of whole grain toast.

Avocado and Tomato Breakfast Sandwich

Preparation Time: 10 minutes

Cooking Time: 5 minutes

Total Time: 15 minutes

Servings: 1

Ingredients:

- 2 slices of whole grain bread
- 1 ripe avocado
- 1 tomato, sliced
- 1-2 slices of cheese (optional)
- Salt and pepper to taste

Directions:

- ➢ Toast the whole grain bread slices to your preferred level of crispiness.
- ➢ While the bread is toasting, halve the avocado, remove the pit, and scoop out the flesh into a bowl. Mash it with a fork and season with salt and pepper.
- ➢ On one side of every slice of toasted bread, spread the mashed avocado.

➤ Layer the tomato slices on top of the mashed avocado on one slice of bread.

➤ If using cheese, place the cheese slices on top of the tomato slices.

➤ Top with the other slice of bread, avocado side down, to make a sandwich.

➤ Optionally, warm the sandwich in a skillet for a minute on each side to melt the cheese and heat through the sandwich.

➤ Cut the sandwich in half diagonally and serve immediately.

Quinoa Breakfast Bowl

Preparation Time: 10 minutes

Cooking Time: 15 minutes (for quinoa)

Total Time: 25 minutes

Servings: 2

Ingredients:

- 1 cup cooked quinoa
- 1 cup mixed berries (blueberries, strawberries, raspberries)
- 1/4 cup chopped nuts (almonds, walnuts, or pecans)
- 2 tablespoons honey or maple syrup
- 1/2 cup Greek yogurt
- Optional: sliced bananas or other favorite fruits

Directions:

- ➢ Prepare quinoa according to package instructions (usually a 1:2 ratio of quinoa to water, simmered for 15 minutes).
- ➢ Divide the cooked quinoa between two bowls.
- ➢ Top each bowl of quinoa with mixed berries, chopped nuts, and sliced bananas or other favorite fruits if desired.
- ➢ Drizzle honey or maple syrup over the bowls for sweetness.
- ➢ Add a dollop of Greek yogurt to each bowl.
- ➢ Serve immediately and mix the ingredients together when ready to eat.

Whole Grain French Toast

Preparation Time: 10 minutes

Cooking Time: 10 minutes

Total Time: 20 minutes

Servings: 2-3

Ingredients:

- 4 slices whole grain bread
- 2 large eggs
- 1/2 cup milk (dairy or plant-based)
- 1 teaspoon vanilla extract
- 1/2 teaspoon ground cinnamon
- Cooking spray or butter for greasing
- Optional toppings: Fresh berries, sliced bananas, maple syrup

Directions:

➢ In a shallow bowl, whisk together eggs, milk, vanilla extract, and cinnamon until well combined.

➢ Grease a non-stick pan or griddle with butter or frying spray before heating it to medium heat.

➢ Dip each slice of whole grain bread into the egg mixture, coating both sides evenly.

- ➤ Place the coated bread slices onto the preheated skillet or griddle.
- ➤ Cook the French toast for about 2-3 minutes on each side, or until golden brown and cooked through.
- ➤ Proceed with the remaining slices of bread.
- ➤ Serve the whole grain French toast warm, topped with fresh berries, sliced bananas, and a drizzle of maple syrup if desired.

Turkey Sausage & Veggie Frittata

Preparation Time: 15 minutes

Cooking Time: 20 minutes

Total Time: 35 minutes

Servings: 4

Ingredients:

- 8 large eggs
- 1/2 cup diced turkey sausage (cooked)
- 1/2 cup diced bell peppers (any color)
- 1/2 cup diced onions
- 1/2 cup chopped spinach or kale
- 1/2 cup shredded cheese (cheddar or mozzarella)
- 1 tablespoon olive oil
- Salt and pepper to taste

Directions:

- ➢ Preheat the oven to 350°F (175°C).
- ➢ In a mixing bowl, whisk together eggs, salt, and pepper until well combined.
- ➢ In a skillet that is oven-safe, warm the olive oil over medium heat.

- ➢ Add diced onions and bell peppers to the skillet and sauté until softened, about 3-4 minutes.
- ➢ Add diced turkey sausage and chopped spinach or kale to the skillet, and cook for an additional 2 minutes.
- ➢ Pour the whisked eggs into the skillet over the sausage and vegetables.
- ➢ Evenly distribute shredded cheese on top of the frittata.
- ➢ Once the oven is hot, place the skillet inside and bake for fifteen to twenty minutes, up to when the frittata is set in the middle.
- ➢ Remove from the oven, let it cool slightly, then slice and serve.

Coconut Milk Chia Pudding with Berries

Preparation Time: 5 minutes (plus chilling time)

Total Time: 4 hours (chilling time)

Servings: 2

Ingredients:

- 1/4 cup chia seeds
- 1 cup coconut milk
- 1 tablespoon maple syrup or honey
- 1/2 teaspoon vanilla extract
- 1/2 cup mixed berries (blueberries, raspberries, strawberries)
- Optional toppings: Shredded coconut, sliced almonds

Directions:

➤ In a bowl, mix together chia seeds, coconut milk, maple syrup (or honey), and vanilla extract.

➤ Make sure the chia seeds are dispersed evenly by giving it a good stir.

➤ After putting the bowl in the refrigerator for 4 hours or overnight, cover it to let the chia seeds absorb the liquid and solidify into a pudding-like consistency.

- ➢ Before serving, stir the chia pudding to ensure it's well combined and smooth.
- ➢ Transfer your chia pudding into glasses or bowls for serving.
- ➢ Top the pudding with mixed berries, shredded coconut, sliced almonds, or your desired toppings.
- ➢ Serve chilled and enjoy this creamy coconut milk chia pudding with a burst of fresh berries!

Smoked Salmon & Avocado Scramble

Preparation Time: 10 minutes

Cooking Time: 5 minutes

Total Time: 15 minutes

Servings: 2

Ingredients:

- 4 large eggs
- 4 oz smoked salmon, chopped
- 1 ripe avocado, diced
- 2 tablespoons chopped fresh dill (optional)
- 1 tablespoon butter or olive oil
- Salt and pepper to taste
- Optional: Sliced whole grain toast

Directions:

➢ Crack the eggs into a bowl, add a pinch of salt and pepper, and whisk them until well combined.

➢ Use a saucepan over medium heat to melt butter or olive oil.

➢ Add the beaten eggs to the skillet and cook, stirring gently, until they start to set but are still slightly runny.

➢ Add chopped smoked salmon to the eggs and continue cooking for another minute, stirring occasionally.

- ➤ Gently fold in diced avocado and chopped fresh dill (if using) into the egg mixture.
- ➤ Cook for an additional 1-2 minutes until the eggs are fully cooked and the avocado is warmed through.
- ➤ Divide the smoked salmon and avocado scramble onto plates.
- ➤ Serve immediately, optionally with slices of whole grain toast.

Avocado and Tomato Breakfast Sandwich

Preparation Time: 10 minutes

Cooking Time: 5 minutes

Total Time: 15 minutes

Servings: 1

Ingredients:

- 2 slices of whole grain bread
- 1 ripe avocado
- 1 tomato, sliced
- 1-2 slices of cheese (optional)
- Salt and pepper to taste

Directions:

➤ Toast the whole grain bread slices to your preferred level of crispiness.

➤ While the bread is toasting, halve the avocado, remove the pit, and scoop out the flesh into a bowl. Mash it with a fork and season with salt and pepper.

➤ On one side of every slice of toasted bread, spread the mashed avocado.

- ➤ Layer the tomato slices on top of the mashed avocado on one slice of bread.
- ➤ If using cheese, place the cheese slices on top of the tomato slices.
- ➤ Top with the other slice of bread, avocado side down, to make a sandwich.
- ➤ Optionally, warm the sandwich in a skillet for a minute on each side to melt the cheese and heat through the sandwich.
- ➤ Cut the sandwich in half diagonally and serve immediately.

Lunch Recipes

Mediterranean Chicken Salad

Preparation Time: 15 minutes
Cooking Time: 15 minutes
Total Time: 30 minutes
Servings: 4

Ingredients:

- • 2 boneless, skinless chicken breasts
- • 1 cup cherry tomatoes, halved
- • 1 cucumber, diced

- 1/2 red onion, thinly sliced

- 1/3 cup Kalamata olives, pitted and halved

- 1/4 cup crumbled feta cheese

- 3 tablespoons extra-virgin olive oil

- 2 tablespoons red wine vinegar

- 1 teaspoon dried oregano

- Salt and pepper to taste

- Fresh parsley for garnish

Directions:

- ➤ Preheat the grill or skillet over medium-high heat.
- ➤ Season the chicken breasts with salt, pepper, and dried oregano.
- ➤ Grill or cook the chicken breasts for about 6-7 minutes per side or until they reach an internal temperature of 165°F (74°C). Before slicing, let them five minutes to rest.
- ➤ In a large mixing bowl, combine cherry tomatoes, diced cucumber, sliced red onion, and Kalamata olives.
- ➤ In a small bowl, whisk together extra-virgin olive oil, red wine vinegar, salt, and pepper to make the dressing.
- ➤ Add the sliced chicken to the vegetable mixture, then drizzle the dressing over the salad. Toss gently to combine.
- ➤ Sprinkle crumbled feta cheese over the top of the salad.
- ➤ Garnish with fresh parsley and serve the Mediterranean chicken salad immediately

Whole Grain Tuna Salad Sandwich

Preparation Time: 10 minutes

Total Time: 10 minutes

Servings: 2

Ingredients:

- 1 can (5 oz) tuna, drained
- 1/4 cup diced red onion
- 1/4 cup diced celery
- 1/4 cup diced red bell pepper
- 2 tablespoons chopped fresh parsley
- 2 tablespoons mayonnaise
- 1 tablespoon lemon juice
- Salt and pepper to taste
- 4 slices whole grain bread
- Lettuce leaves, tomato slices (optional, for serving)

Directions:

- ➢ In a mixing bowl, combine the drained tuna, diced red onion, diced celery, diced red bell pepper, and chopped parsley.
- ➢ Add mayonnaise and lemon juice to the tuna mixture. Blend until all components are thoroughly blended.

- ➢ Add salt and pepper to taste when preparing the tuna salad. As desired, adjust the seasoning.
- ➢ Toast the slices of whole grain bread (optional).
- ➢ Divide the tuna salad evenly among two slices of bread.
- ➢ Top with lettuce leaves, tomato slices, if using, and cover with the remaining slices of bread.
- ➢ Serve immediately and enjoy your whole grain tuna salad sandwich!

Mediterranean Veggie Pita

Preparation Time: 15 minutes

Total Time: 15 minutes

Servings: 2

Ingredients:

- 2 whole wheat pita bread rounds
- 1 cup mixed salad greens (lettuce, spinach, arugula)
- 1/2 cup diced cucumber
- 1/2 cup cherry tomatoes, halved
- 1/4 cup sliced red onion
- 1/4 cup sliced Kalamata olives
- 1/4 cup crumbled feta cheese
- 2 tablespoons chopped fresh parsley
- 2 tablespoons extra-virgin olive oil
- 1 tablespoon red wine vinegar
- Salt and pepper to taste
- Hummus for spreading (optional)

Directions:

➢ In a mixing bowl, combine mixed salad greens, diced cucumber, halved cherry tomatoes, sliced red onion, sliced Kalamata olives, crumbled feta cheese, and chopped parsley.

➢ In a small bowl, whisk together extra-virgin olive oil, red wine vinegar, salt, and pepper to create the dressing.

➢ Pour the dressing over the vegetable mixture and toss gently to coat all ingredients.

➢ Warm the whole wheat pita bread rounds slightly in a toaster or microwave.

➢ If desired, spread hummus on the inside of the pita bread rounds.

➢ Stuff the pita pockets with the Mediterranean veggie salad mixture.

➢ Serve immediately and enjoy your flavorful Mediterranean veggie pita!

Grilled Chicken Caesar Salad with Avocado

Preparation Time: 15 minutes

Cooking Time: 15 minutes

Total Time: 30 minutes

Servings: 4

Ingredients:

For the Salad:

- 2 boneless, skinless chicken breasts
- 1 head romaine lettuce, washed and chopped
- 1 avocado, sliced
- 1/4 cup shaved or grated Parmesan cheese
- Croutons (store-bought or homemade)

For the Caesar Dressing:

- 1/2 cup mayonnaise
- 2 tablespoons freshly squeezed lemon juice
- 2 cloves garlic, minced
- 2 anchovy fillets (optional), minced or anchovy paste
- 1 teaspoon Dijon mustard
- 1/4 cup grated Parmesan cheese
- Salt and black pepper to taste

> ➢ 2 tablespoons olive oil

Directions:

➢ Preheat the grill over medium-high heat.

➢ Season the chicken breasts with salt and pepper, then grill for about 6-7 minutes per side until cooked through. Before slicing, let them a few minutes to rest.

➢ In a large bowl, toss the chopped romaine lettuce with avocado slices, Parmesan cheese, and croutons.

➢ For the Caesar dressing, in a separate bowl, whisk together mayonnaise, lemon juice, minced garlic, anchovy fillets or paste, Dijon mustard, grated Parmesan cheese, salt, and pepper. Add olive oil gradually and whisk until fully blended.

➢ To the salad bowl, add the grilled chicken slices.

➢ Drizzle the Caesar dressing over the salad or serve it on the side.

➢ Toss the salad gently to coat evenly with the dressing.

➢ Serve the Grilled Chicken Caesar Salad immediately.

Lentil Soup with Whole Wheat Bread

Preparation Time: 15 minutes

Cooking Time: 45 minutes

Total Time: 1 hour

Servings: 4

Ingredients:

- 1 cup rinsed and drained dried lentils, either brown or green
- 1 onion, chopped
- 2 carrots, diced
- 2 celery stalks, diced
- 3 cloves garlic, minced
- 4 cups vegetable or chicken broth
- 1 can (14 oz) diced tomatoes
- 1 teaspoon dried thyme
- 1 teaspoon dried oregano
- 1 bay leaf
- Salt and pepper to taste
- Fresh parsley for garnish
- Whole wheat bread slices for serving

Directions:

➢ Place the olive oil in a large pot and heat it to medium.

- Add chopped onion, diced carrots, and diced celery. Cook for about 5 minutes until vegetables soften.
- Stir in minced garlic and cook for an additional minute until fragrant.
- Add dried lentils, vegetable or chicken broth, diced tomatoes (with their juices), dried thyme, dried oregano, bay leaf, salt, and pepper to the pot.
- After bringing the mixture to a boil, turn down the heat. Cover the pot and let it simmer for about 30-35 minutes or until the lentils are tender.
- Once the lentils are cooked, remove the bay leaf from the soup.
- Taste and adjust seasoning if needed.
- Ladle the lentil soup into bowls, garnish with fresh parsley, and serve with slices of whole wheat bread.

Mediterranean Hummus Plate

Preparation Time: 10 minutes

Total Time: 10 minutes

Servings: 2

Ingredients:

- 1 cup hummus (store-bought or homemade)
- 1/2 cup cherry tomatoes, halved
- 1/2 cucumber, sliced
- 1/4 cup Kalamata olives
- 1/4 cup crumbled feta cheese
- 2 tablespoons extra-virgin olive oil
- 1 tablespoon chopped fresh parsley
- Pita bread or pita chips for serving

Directions:

➢ Spread the hummus evenly on a serving plate.

➢ Arrange cherry tomatoes, cucumber slices, and Kalamata olives on top of the hummus.

➢ Sprinkle crumbled feta cheese over the vegetables.

➢ Drizzle extra-virgin olive oil over the hummus plate.

➢ Garnish with chopped fresh parsley.

➢ Accompany with pita chips or pita bread for dipping.

Quinoa and Chickpea Salad

Preparation Time: 15 minutes

Cooking Time: 15 minutes

Total Time: 30 minutes

Servings: 4

Ingredients:

- 1 cup quinoa, rinsed
- 2 cups water or vegetable broth
- Quinoa, rinsed and drained, in one can (15 oz).
- 1 red bell pepper, diced
- 1/2 English cucumber, diced
- 1/4 cup chopped fresh parsley
- 1/4 cup chopped fresh mint (optional)
- 1/4 cup crumbled feta cheese (optional)
- 2 tablespoons extra-virgin olive oil
- 2 tablespoons lemon juice
- Salt and pepper to taste

Directions:

➤ In a medium saucepan, bring water or vegetable broth to a boil. Add quinoa, reduce heat to low, cover, and simmer for

15 minutes or until quinoa is cooked and liquid is absorbed. Once the heat is off, let it cool.

➢ In a large mixing bowl, combine cooked quinoa, drained chickpeas, diced red bell pepper, diced cucumber, chopped parsley, and chopped mint (if using).

➢ Pour lemon juice and extra virgin olive oil over the salad. Toss gently to combine.

➢ Season with salt and pepper according to taste.

➢ If desired, sprinkle crumbled feta cheese on top before serving.

Phase 3 Dinner Recipes

Whole Grain Spaghetti with Turkey Meatballs

Preparation Time: 20 minutes

Cooking Time: 25 minutes

Total Time: 45 minutes

Servings: 4

Ingredients:

For Turkey Meatballs:

- 1 pound ground turkey
- 1/4 cup breadcrumbs (whole grain)
- 1/4 cup grated Parmesan cheese
- 1 egg
- 2 cloves garlic, minced
- 2 tablespoons chopped parsley
- Salt and black pepper to taste
- Olive oil for cooking

For Spaghetti:

- 8 oz whole grain spaghetti
- 2 cups marinara sauce (store-bought or homemade)

- Chopped fresh basil for garnish

Directions:

➤ In a bowl, combine ground turkey, breadcrumbs, grated Parmesan, egg, minced garlic, chopped parsley, salt, and pepper. Mix well and form into meatballs.

➤ In a large skillet over a medium-high flame, warm the olive oil. Cook meatballs for about 8-10 minutes until browned and cooked through.

➤ Meanwhile, cook whole grain spaghetti according to package instructions. Drain.

➤ Warm marinara sauce in a saucepan. Add cooked meatballs to the sauce and let them simmer together for a few minutes.

➤ Serve the turkey meatballs and marinara sauce over the cooked whole grain spaghetti. Garnish with chopped fresh basil.

Black Bean Burgers on Whole Wheat Buns

Preparation Time: 20 minutes

Cooking Time: 10 minutes

Total Time: 30 minutes

Servings: 4

Ingredients:

For Black Bean Burgers:

- Two cans (15 oz each) of rinsed and drained black beans
- 1/2 cup breadcrumbs (whole wheat)
- 1/4 cup finely chopped onion
- 2 cloves garlic, minced
- 1 teaspoon ground cumin
- 1 teaspoon chili powder
- 1/4 cup chopped cilantro
- Salt and pepper to taste
- Olive oil for cooking

For Serving:

- 4 whole wheat burger buns
- Lettuce leaves, tomato slices, avocado (optional)

- Condiments of choice (ketchup, mustard, mayo)

Directions:

- ➢ In a bowl, mash black beans with a fork or potato masher until mostly smooth but still chunky.
- ➢ Add breadcrumbs, finely chopped onion, minced garlic, ground cumin, chili powder, chopped cilantro, salt, and pepper to the mashed beans. Mix until well combined.
- ➢ Separate the mixture into four equal parts and form each part into a patty.
- ➢ In a large skillet over a medium-low flame, warm the olive oil. Cook black bean patties for about 4-5 minutes per side until browned and heated through.
- ➢ Toast whole wheat burger buns if desired. Assemble the burgers with lettuce leaves, tomato slices, avocado (if using), black bean patty, and your choice of condiments.

Mediterranean Chicken Skewers with Tzatziki

Preparation Time: 20 minutes

Cooking Time: 10 minutes

Total Time: 30 minutes

Servings: 4

Ingredients:

For Chicken Skewers:

- One and a half pounds of cubed, skinless, boneless chicken breasts
- 1 red bell pepper, cut into chunks
- 1 yellow bell pepper, cut into chunks
- 1 red onion, cut into chunks
- 2 tablespoons olive oil
- 2 teaspoons dried oregano
- 1 teaspoon paprika
- Salt and pepper to taste
- Wooden skewers (pre-soaked in water for 20-30 minutes)

For Tzatziki Sauce:

- 1 cup Greek yogurt

- 1 cucumber, grated and drained
- 2 cloves garlic, minced
- 1 tablespoon chopped fresh dill
- 1 tablespoon lemon juice
- Salt and pepper to taste

Directions:

➢ In a bowl, combine cubed chicken, bell peppers, red onion, olive oil, dried oregano, paprika, salt, and pepper. After thoroughly mixing, let it marinade for 15 to 20 minutes.

➢ Make the tzatziki sauce while the chicken marinates. In another bowl, combine Greek yogurt, grated and drained cucumber, minced garlic, chopped fresh dill, lemon juice, salt, and pepper. Mix thoroughly and refrigerate until serving.

➢ Thread marinated chicken, bell peppers, and red onion onto the pre-soaked wooden skewers.

➢ Turn the heat up to medium-high on the grill or grill pan. Grill the chicken skewers for about 4-5 minutes on each side until the chicken is cooked through and veggies are slightly charred.

➢ Serve the Mediterranean chicken skewers with tzatziki sauce on the side for dipping.

Spaghetti Squash Pad Thai

Preparation Time: 15 minutes

Cooking Time: 30 minutes

Total Time: 45 minutes

Servings: 4

Ingredients:

- 1 medium spaghetti squash
- 2 tablespoons olive oil
- 2 cloves garlic, minced
- 1 red bell pepper, thinly sliced
- 1 cup shredded carrots
- 1 cup bean sprouts
- 2 green onions, thinly sliced
- 2 eggs, beaten
- 1/4 cup chopped peanuts (optional)
- Fresh cilantro for garnish

For Pad Thai Sauce:

- ➤ 3 tablespoons soy sauce (or tamari for gluten-free)
- ➤ 2 tablespoons fish sauce (optional for non-vegetarian)
- ➤ 2 tablespoons rice vinegar
- ➤ 2 tablespoons brown sugar (or honey)

- ➤ Juice of 1 lime
- ➤ 1 teaspoon Sriracha sauce (adjust to taste)
- ➤ 1/4 cup chopped fresh cilantro

Directions:

- ➤ Preheat the oven to 400°F (200°C). Cut the spaghetti squash in half lengthwise, and then remove the seeds. Season the interior with salt, pepper, and olive oil. Arrange the halves on a baking sheet, face down.
- ➤ Bake for 30-40 minutes until the squash is tender. Let it cool for a few minutes, then scrape the flesh with a fork to create "spaghetti."
- ➤ Mix all of the ingredients for the Pad Thai sauce in a small bowl. Adjust the seasoning to your preference.
- ➤ In a big skillet or wok, heat the olive oil over medium-high heat. Cook the minced garlic for 30 seconds, or until it becomes aromatic.
- ➤ Add sliced red bell pepper and shredded carrots to the skillet. Stir-fry for 2-3 minutes until slightly softened.
- ➤ After pushing the veggies to one side of the skillet, cover the empty side with the beaten eggs. After the eggs are cooked, scramble them and combine them with the vegetables.
- ➤ Add the spaghetti squash "noodles" to the skillet along with bean sprouts and green onions. Pour the Pad Thai sauce over the mixture. Mix everything together until thoroughly hot and properly mixed.
- ➤ Serve the Spaghetti Squash Pad Thai garnished with chopped peanuts (if using) and fresh cilantro.

Mediterranean Stuffed Portobello Mushrooms

Preparation Time: 20 minutes

Cooking Time: 20 minutes

Total Time: 40 minutes

Servings: 4

Ingredients:

- 4 large Portobello mushrooms, stems removed and cleaned
- 1 cup cooked quinoa or couscous
- One can (14.2 oz) of drained and diced artichoke hearts
- 1 cup cherry tomatoes, halved
- 1/2 cup crumbled feta cheese
- 2 tablespoons chopped fresh basil
- 2 tablespoons chopped fresh parsley
- 2 cloves garlic, minced
- 2 tablespoons olive oil
- Salt and pepper to taste

Directions:

➢ Preheat the oven to 375°F (190°C). Line a baking sheet with parchment paper.

- In a bowl, mix together cooked quinoa or couscous, chopped artichoke hearts, halved cherry tomatoes, crumbled feta cheese, chopped fresh basil, chopped fresh parsley, minced garlic, olive oil, salt, and pepper.
- Place the Portobello mushrooms on the prepared baking sheet, cap side down. Drizzle a little olive oil on the mushrooms and season with salt and pepper.
- Spoon the quinoa (or couscous) mixture into the Portobello mushrooms, dividing it equally among them and pressing gently.
- Bake in the preheated oven for about 18-20 minutes or until the mushrooms are tender and the filling is heated through.
- Before serving, take them out of the oven and allow them to cool for a few minutes.

Coconut Curry Cauliflower Rice with Shrimp

Preparation Time: 15 minutes

Cooking Time: 15 minutes

Total Time: 30 minutes

Servings: 4

Ingredients:

- 1 pound shrimp, peeled and deveined
- 1 medium head cauliflower, grated or riced
- 1 red bell pepper, diced
- 1 cup snow peas, trimmed
- 1 can (14 oz) coconut milk
- 2 tablespoons red curry paste
- 2 tablespoons soy sauce
- 2 tablespoons lime juice
- 2 cloves garlic, minced
- 2 tablespoons chopped fresh cilantro
- 2 tablespoons olive oil
- Salt and pepper to taste

Directions:

- In a big skillet or wok, warm up the olive oil over medium heat. Cook the minced garlic for 30 seconds, or until it becomes aromatic.
- Add diced red bell pepper and trimmed snow peas to the skillet. Stir-fry for two to three minutes, or until tender.
- Push the vegetables to the side of the skillet and add the shrimp. Shrimp should be cooked for 2 to 3 minutes on each side, or until they become opaque and pink. Take out and reserve the shrimp.
- In the same skillet, add grated cauliflower and stir-fry for 3-4 minutes until it begins to soften.
- In a small bowl, whisk together coconut milk, red curry paste, soy sauce, and lime juice.
- Pour the coconut curry mixture into the skillet with cauliflower rice. Stir well to combine.
- Return the cooked shrimp to the skillet and toss everything together until heated through.
- Season with salt and pepper according to taste.
- Garnish with chopped fresh cilantro before serving.

Stir-fried Broccoli and Beef with Ginger

Preparation Time: 15 minutes

Cooking Time: 15 minutes

Total Time: 30 minutes

Servings: 4

Ingredients:

- One pound of finely sliced beef flank or sirloin
- 4 cups broccoli florets
- 1 red bell pepper, thinly sliced
- 2 cloves garlic, minced
- 1 tablespoon fresh ginger, grated
- 3 tablespoons soy sauce
- 2 tablespoons oyster sauce
- 1 tablespoon sesame oil
- 2 tablespoons vegetable oil
- Sesame seeds for garnish (optional)
- Cooked brown rice for serving

Directions:

- In a bowl, combine thinly sliced beef with minced garlic, grated ginger, soy sauce, and oyster sauce. Toss well to coat the beef and let it marinate for 10-15 minutes.
- Heat vegetable oil in a large skillet or wok over high heat. Add marinated beef to the skillet and stir-fry for 2-3 minutes until browned. After taking the steak out of the griddle, set it aside.
- If necessary, add a little extra oil to the same skillet. Stir-fry broccoli florets and sliced red bell pepper for 3-4 minutes until they are crisp-tender.
- Return the cooked beef to the skillet and toss everything together.
- Drizzle sesame oil over the stir-fry and toss again to combine.
- Garnish with sesame seeds if desired.
- Serve the Stir-fried Broccoli and Beef with Ginger over cooked brown rice.

Salmon with Mango Salsa

Preparation Time: 15 minutes

Cooking Time: 10 minutes

Total Time: 25 minutes

Servings: 4

Ingredients:

- Four 6-ounce salmon fillets, either skin-on or skinless
- 2 ripe mangoes, peeled and diced
- 1/2 red bell pepper, diced
- 1/2 red onion, finely chopped
- 1 jalapeño, seeded and minced
- Juice of 2 limes
- 2 tablespoons chopped fresh cilantro
- 1 tablespoon olive oil
- Salt and pepper to taste

Directions:

➢ In a bowl, combine diced mangoes, diced red bell pepper, finely chopped red onion, minced jalapeño, lime juice, chopped cilantro, olive oil, salt, and pepper to make the mango salsa. Mix well and refrigerate until serving.

- Preheat the oven to 400°F (200°C). Line a baking sheet with parchment paper.
- Pat dry the salmon fillets with paper towels. Use salt and pepper to season both sides.
- After the baking sheet is ready, put the salmon fillets on it.
- Bake the salmon in the preheated oven for about 8-10 minutes until cooked through or until desired doneness.
- Once cooked, remove the salmon from the oven.
- Serve the baked salmon topped with the refreshing mango salsa.

Phase Three Meal Plan

Here's a two-week meal plan structure incorporating the provided Phase Three recipes for breakfast, lunch, and dinner in the South Beach Diet:

Week 1:

Day 1:

Breakfast: Greek Yogurt with Berries and Almonds

Lunch: Mediterranean Chicken Salad

Dinner: Whole Grain Spaghetti with Turkey Meatballs

Day 2:

Breakfast: Spinach and Feta Omelet

Lunch: Whole Grain Tuna Salad Sandwich

Dinner: Black Bean Burgers on Whole Wheat Buns

Day 3:

Breakfast: Avocado and Tomato Breakfast Sandwich

Lunch: Mediterranean Veggie Pita

Dinner: Mediterranean Chicken Skewers with Tzatziki

Day 4:

Breakfast: Quinoa Breakfast Bowl

Lunch: Grilled Chicken Caesar Salad with Avocado

Dinner: Spaghetti Squash Pad Thai

Day 5:

Breakfast: Whole Grain French Toast

Lunch: Lentil Soup with Whole Wheat Bread

Dinner: Mediterranean Stuffed Portobello Mushrooms

Day 6:

Breakfast: Turkey Sausage & Veggie Frittata

Lunch: Mediterranean Hummus Plate

Dinner: Seared Tuna Steaks with Cucumber Avocado Salsa

Day 7:

Breakfast: Coconut Milk Chia Pudding with Berries

Lunch: Quinoa and Chickpea Salad

Dinner: Coconut Curry Cauliflower Rice with Shrimp

Week 2:

Day 8:

Breakfast: Smoked Salmon & Avocado Scramble

Lunch: Mediterranean Chicken Salad

Dinner: Stir-fried Broccoli and Beef with Ginger

Day 9:

Breakfast: Avocado and Tomato Breakfast Sandwich

Lunch: Whole Grain Tuna Salad Sandwich

Dinner: Salmon with Mango Salsa

Day 10:

Breakfast: Greek Yogurt with Berries and Almonds

Lunch: Mediterranean Veggie Pita

Dinner: Whole Grain Spaghetti with Turkey Meatballs

Day 11:

Breakfast: Quinoa Breakfast Bowl

Lunch: Grilled Chicken Caesar Salad with Avocado

Dinner: Black Bean Burgers on Whole Wheat Buns

Day 12:

Breakfast: Coconut Milk Chia Pudding with Berries

Lunch: Lentil Soup with Whole Wheat Bread

Dinner: Mediterranean Chicken Skewers with Tzatziki

Day 13:

Breakfast: Spinach and Feta Omelet

Lunch: Mediterranean Hummus Plate

Dinner: Spaghetti Squash Pad Thai

Day 14:

Breakfast: Turkey Sausage & Veggie Frittata

Lunch: Quinoa and Chickpea Salad

Dinner: Seared Tuna Steaks with Cucumber Avocado Salsa

This meal plan provides a diverse selection of Phase Three recipes for breakfast, lunch, and dinner, incorporating a variety of whole grains, lean proteins, and vegetables in alignment with the South Beach Diet principles. Feel free to adjust portions and ingredients according to personal preferences and dietary needs.

Snack Suggestions

Snack suggestions include a mix of Phase Two snacks with an emphasis on portion control and healthier choices. Options may include nuts, Greek yogurt, fresh fruits, vegetable sticks with hummus, or homemade energy bars.

Strategies for Long-Term Success and Health Maintenance

Consistency: Establish a routine that includes regular, balanced meals and snacks.

Physical Activity: Continue incorporating regular exercise into daily life for overall fitness and health.

Mindful Eating Practices: Listen to your body's hunger and fullness cues to prevent overeating.

Stress Management: Adopt stress-relieving techniques like meditation, yoga, or hobbies to maintain mental health.

Regular Check-ins: Periodically assess progress and make adjustments as needed to maintain goals.

Support System: Surround yourself with a supportive network to stay motivated and accountable.

Celebrating Milestones: Acknowledge and celebrate achievements to stay motivated and positive.

This Phase Three breakdown provides a thorough guide to entering a maintenance phase, emphasizing strategies for maintaining overall health and long-term success in accordance with the South Beach Diet's tenets, as well as balanced meal planning, snack ideas, and lifelong healthy eating habits.

Conclusion

Congratulations on finishing the South Beach Diet and accomplishing your goal! As you've moved through the program's several phases, you've not only lost weight but also started down the road to long-term lifestyle and health improvements.

Honoring Significant Occasions

It's important to recognize and commemorate the victories you've had while following the South Beach Diet. Whether you've lost weight, made healthier food choices, or found more energy, give yourself a time to acknowledge and enjoy your successes. Celebrating accomplishments can serve as a source of inspiration and support for ongoing achievement.

Considering Achievement

Give yourself some time to consider the accomplishments you've made. Think on how your body, mind, and general well-being have improved. Maybe you've gained a better grasp of nutrition, learned how to prepare meals and make healthier food choices, or even tried new dishes. Acknowledge these successes since they are essential steps on the path to long-term wellness.

Creating New Objectives

As this phase of the South Beach Diet comes to an end, think about establishing new objectives for your wellbeing. These objectives could be preserving your current weight, advancing your weight loss efforts, or emphasizing other wellness-related objectives like boosting physical activity, reducing stress, or enhancing sleep. You'll remain inspired and dedicated to your health journey if you set reasonable and doable goals for yourself.

Including Long-Term Routines

You now have important understanding about nutrition, portion control, and balanced eating practices thanks to the South Beach Diet. It's time to apply these lessons to your everyday life going forward. Maintain your conscious eating habits, physical activity level, and self-care routine. Recall that maintaining good habits consistently is essential for long-term success.

Concluding Remarks on Long-Term Health and Weight Control

Prolonged well-being and managing weight do not require band-aids or short-term cures. Rather, they focus on developing a well-rounded way of life where eating healthily, exercising, controlling stress, and getting enough sleep are all important.

Adopting a Comprehensive Perspective

It's critical to take a holistic approach to health, which includes social, mental, and emotional well-being in addition to food decisions. Managing stress, practicing mindfulness, self-care, and cultivating positive connections are all essential to preserving general wellbeing.

Proceeding Forward

Recall that your quest for ideal health is a continuous process as you move past the South Beach Diet's set phases. Remain devoted to the healthy routines you've established, conscious of the decisions you make, and flexible in response to life's changes. Accept your new way of living as a rewarding and long-term approach to enhance your health and wellbeing.

WEIGHT LOSS TRACKER & 30-DAYS WELLNESS TRACKER

Thank you for being a part of this journey. I congratulate you and I also appreciate you for taking a bold step by getting a copy of the South Beach Diet Book for 2024.

As a little token to show my appreciation for your purchase, here's your bonus and I hope you love it and use it to track your weight loss journey

You can do well to drop positive feedback and tell me what you think of the book in the Amazon book review section.

Thanks, my friend!

The South Beach Diet
Measurement Tracker

Weight _____   Weight _____

Date _____   Date _____

RIGHT ARM _____ _____ RIGHT ARM

LEFT ARM _____ _____ LEFT ARM

CGEST _____ _____ CGEST

WAIST _____ _____ WAIST

HIPS _____ _____ HIPS

RIGHT THIGH _____ _____ RIGHT THIGH

LEFT THIGH _____ _____ LEFT THIGH

RIGHT CALF _____ _____ RIGHT CALF

LEFT CALF _____ _____ LEFT CALF

NOTES
•
•

The South Beach Diet
Measurement Tracker

BEFORE   **AFTER**

Weight _____   Weight _____

Date _____   Date _____

BEFORE		AFTER
RIGHT ARM _____		_____ RIGHT ARM
LEFT ARM _____		_____ LEFT ARM
CGEST _____		_____ CGEST
WAIST _____		_____ WAIST
HIPS _____		_____ HIPS
RIGHT THIGH _____		_____ RIGHT THIGH
LEFT THIGH _____		_____ LEFT THIGH
RIGHT CALF _____		_____ RIGHT CALF
LEFT CALF _____		_____ LEFT CALF

NOTES

-
-

The South Beach Diet
Measurement Tracker

Weight _____   Weight _____

Date _____   Date _____

RIGHT ARM _____   _____ RIGHT ARM

LEFT ARM _____   _____ LEFT ARM

CGEST _____   _____ CGEST

WAIST _____   _____ WAIST

HIPS _____   _____ HIPS

RIGHT THIGH _____   _____ RIGHT THIGH

LEFT THIGH _____   _____ LEFT THIGH

RIGHT CALF _____   _____ RIGHT CALF

LEFT CALF _____   _____ LEFT CALF

NOTES
•
•

The South Beach Diet
Measurement Tracker

BEFORE	AFTER

Weight _____   **Weight** _____

Date _____   **Date** _____

RIGHT ARM _____	_____ RIGHT ARM

LEFT ARM _____   _____ LEFT ARM

CGEST _____   _____ CGEST

WAIST _____   _____ WAIST

HIPS _____   _____ HIPS

RIGHT THIGH _____   _____ RIGHT THIGH

LEFT THIGH _____   _____ LEFT THIGH

RIGHT CALF _____   _____ RIGHT CALF

LEFT CALF _____   _____ LEFT CALF

NOTES

-
-

The South Beach Diet
Measurement Tracker

BEFORE   AFTER

Weight _____   Weight _____

Date _____   Date _____

RIGHT
ARM _____   _____ RIGHT ARM

LEFT
ARM _____   _____ LEFT ARM

CGEST _____   _____ CGEST

WAIST _____   _____ WAIST

HIPS _____   _____ HIPS

RIGHT
THIGH _____   _____ RIGHT THIGH

LEFT
THIGH _____   _____ LEFT THIGH

RIGHT
CALF _____   _____ RIGHT CALF

LEFT
CALF _____   _____ LEFT CALF

NOTES
•
•

The South Beach Diet
Measurement Tracker

BEFORE   AFTER

Weight _____   Weight _____

Date _____   Date _____

RIGHT   RIGHT
ARM   _____   _____   ARM

LEFT   LEFT
ARM   _____   _____   ARM

CGEST _____   _____   CGEST

WAIST _____   _____   WAIST

HIPS _____   _____   HIPS

RIGHT   RIGHT
THIGH _____   _____   THIGH

LEFT   LEFT
THIGH _____   _____   THIGH

RIGHT   RIGHT
CALF _____   _____   CALF

LEFT   LEFT
CALF _____   _____   CALF

NOTES

-
-

30 Day Wellness Tracker

MONTH: _____

SLEEP

DAY 1	DAY 2	DAY 3	DAY 4	DAY 5	DAY 6	DAY 7	DAY 8	DAY 9	DAY 10
DAY 11	DAY 12	DAY 13	DAY 14	DAY 15	DAY 16	DAY 17	DAY 18	DAY 19	DAY 20
DAY 21	DAY 22	DAY 23	DAY 24	DAY 25	DAY 26	DAY 27	DAY 28	DAY 29	DAY 30

SELF CARE ROUTINE

DAY 1	DAY 2	DAY 3	DAY 4	DAY 5	DAY 6	DAY 7	DAY 8	DAY 9	DAY 10
DAY 11	DAY 12	DAY 13	DAY 14	DAY 15	DAY 16	DAY 17	DAY 18	DAY 19	DAY 20
DAY 21	DAY 22	DAY 23	DAY 24	DAY 25	DAY 26	DAY 27	DAY 28	DAY 29	DAY 30

EXERCISE

DAY 1	DAY 2	DAY 3	DAY 4	DAY 5	DAY 6	DAY 7	DAY 8	DAY 9	DAY 10
DAY 11	DAY 12	DAY 13	DAY 14	DAY 15	DAY 16	DAY 17	DAY 18	DAY 19	DAY 20
DAY 21	DAY 22	DAY 23	DAY 24	DAY 25	DAY 26	DAY 27	DAY 28	DAY 29	DAY 30

MEAL PLAN

DAY 1	DAY 2	DAY 3	DAY 4	DAY 5	DAY 6	DAY 7	DAY 8	DAY 9	DAY 10
DAY 11	DAY 12	DAY 13	DAY 14	DAY 15	DAY 16	DAY 17	DAY 18	DAY 19	DAY 20
DAY 21	DAY 22	DAY 23	DAY 24	DAY 25	DAY 26	DAY 27	DAY 28	DAY 29	DAY 30

30 Day Wellness Tracker

SLEEP

DAY 1	DAY 2	DAY 3	DAY 4	DAY 5	DAY 6	DAY 7	DAY 8	DAY 9	DAY 10
DAY 11	DAY 12	DAY 13	DAY 14	DAY 15	DAY 16	DAY 17	DAY 18	DAY 19	DAY 20
DAY 21	DAY 22	DAY 23	DAY 24	DAY 25	DAY 26	DAY 27	DAY 28	DAY 29	DAY 30

SELF CARE ROUTINE

DAY 1	DAY 2	DAY 3	DAY 4	DAY 5	DAY 6	DAY 7	DAY 8	DAY 9	DAY 10
DAY 11	DAY 12	DAY 13	DAY 14	DAY 15	DAY 16	DAY 17	DAY 18	DAY 19	DAY 20
DAY 21	DAY 22	DAY 23	DAY 24	DAY 25	DAY 26	DAY 27	DAY 28	DAY 29	DAY 30

EXERCISE

DAY 1	DAY 2	DAY 3	DAY 4	DAY 5	DAY 6	DAY 7	DAY 8	DAY 9	DAY 10
DAY 11	DAY 12	DAY 13	DAY 14	DAY 15	DAY 16	DAY 17	DAY 18	DAY 19	DAY 20
DAY 21	DAY 22	DAY 23	DAY 24	DAY 25	DAY 26	DAY 27	DAY 28	DAY 29	DAY 30

MEAL PLAN

DAY 1	DAY 2	DAY 3	DAY 4	DAY 5	DAY 6	DAY 7	DAY 8	DAY 9	DAY 10
DAY 11	DAY 12	DAY 13	DAY 14	DAY 15	DAY 16	DAY 17	DAY 18	DAY 19	DAY 20
DAY 21	DAY 22	DAY 23	DAY 24	DAY 25	DAY 26	DAY 27	DAY 28	DAY 29	DAY 30

30 Day Wellness Tracker

MONTH: _____

SLEEP

DAY 1	DAY 2	DAY 3	DAY 4	DAY 5	DAY 6	DAY 7	DAY 8	DAY 9	DAY 10
DAY 11	DAY 12	DAY 13	DAY 14	DAY 15	DAY 16	DAY 17	DAY 18	DAY 19	DAY 20
DAY 21	DAY 22	DAY 23	DAY 24	DAY 25	DAY 26	DAY 27	DAY 28	DAY 29	DAY 30

SELF CARE ROUTINE

DAY 1	DAY 2	DAY 3	DAY 4	DAY 5	DAY 6	DAY 7	DAY 8	DAY 9	DAY 10
DAY 11	DAY 12	DAY 13	DAY 14	DAY 15	DAY 16	DAY 17	DAY 18	DAY 19	DAY 20
DAY 21	DAY 22	DAY 23	DAY 24	DAY 25	DAY 26	DAY 27	DAY 28	DAY 29	DAY 30

EXERCISE

DAY 1	DAY 2	DAY 3	DAY 4	DAY 5	DAY 6	DAY 7	DAY 8	DAY 9	DAY 10
DAY 11	DAY 12	DAY 13	DAY 14	DAY 15	DAY 16	DAY 17	DAY 18	DAY 19	DAY 20
DAY 21	DAY 22	DAY 23	DAY 24	DAY 25	DAY 26	DAY 27	DAY 28	DAY 29	DAY 30

MEAL PLAN

DAY 1	DAY 2	DAY 3	DAY 4	DAY 5	DAY 6	DAY 7	DAY 8	DAY 9	DAY 10
DAY 11	DAY 12	DAY 13	DAY 14	DAY 15	DAY 16	DAY 17	DAY 18	DAY 19	DAY 20
DAY 21	DAY 22	DAY 23	DAY 24	DAY 25	DAY 26	DAY 27	DAY 28	DAY 29	DAY 30

30 Day Wellness Tracker

MONTH: _____

SLEEP

DAY 1	DAY 2	DAY 3	DAY 4	DAY 5	DAY 6	DAY 7	DAY 8	DAY 9	DAY 10
DAY 11	DAY 12	DAY 13	DAY 14	DAY 15	DAY 16	DAY 17	DAY 18	DAY 19	DAY 20
DAY 21	DAY 22	DAY 23	DAY 24	DAY 25	DAY 26	DAY 27	DAY 28	DAY 29	DAY 30

SELF CARE ROUTINE

DAY 1	DAY 2	DAY 3	DAY 4	DAY 5	DAY 6	DAY 7	DAY 8	DAY 9	DAY 10
DAY 11	DAY 12	DAY 13	DAY 14	DAY 15	DAY 16	DAY 17	DAY 18	DAY 19	DAY 20
DAY 21	DAY 22	DAY 23	DAY 24	DAY 25	DAY 26	DAY 27	DAY 28	DAY 29	DAY 30

EXERCISE

DAY 1	DAY 2	DAY 3	DAY 4	DAY 5	DAY 6	DAY 7	DAY 8	DAY 9	DAY 10
DAY 11	DAY 12	DAY 13	DAY 14	DAY 15	DAY 16	DAY 17	DAY 18	DAY 19	DAY 20
DAY 21	DAY 22	DAY 23	DAY 24	DAY 25	DAY 26	DAY 27	DAY 28	DAY 29	DAY 30

MEAL PLAN

DAY 1	DAY 2	DAY 3	DAY 4	DAY 5	DAY 6	DAY 7	DAY 8	DAY 9	DAY 10
DAY 11	DAY 12	DAY 13	DAY 14	DAY 15	DAY 16	DAY 17	DAY 18	DAY 19	DAY 20
DAY 21	DAY 22	DAY 23	DAY 24	DAY 25	DAY 26	DAY 27	DAY 28	DAY 29	DAY 30

30 Day Wellness Tracker

MONTH: _____

SLEEP

DAY 1	DAY 2	DAY 3	DAY 4	DAY 5	DAY 6	DAY 7	DAY 8	DAY 9	DAY 10
DAY 11	DAY 12	DAY 13	DAY 14	DAY 15	DAY 16	DAY 17	DAY 18	DAY 19	DAY 20
DAY 21	DAY 22	DAY 23	DAY 24	DAY 25	DAY 26	DAY 27	DAY 28	DAY 29	DAY 30

SELF CARE ROUTINE

DAY 1	DAY 2	DAY 3	DAY 4	DAY 5	DAY 6	DAY 7	DAY 8	DAY 9	DAY 10
DAY 11	DAY 12	DAY 13	DAY 14	DAY 15	DAY 16	DAY 17	DAY 18	DAY 19	DAY 20
DAY 21	DAY 22	DAY 23	DAY 24	DAY 25	DAY 26	DAY 27	DAY 28	DAY 29	DAY 30

EXERCISE

DAY 1	DAY 2	DAY 3	DAY 4	DAY 5	DAY 6	DAY 7	DAY 8	DAY 9	DAY 10
DAY 11	DAY 12	DAY 13	DAY 14	DAY 15	DAY 16	DAY 17	DAY 18	DAY 19	DAY 20
DAY 21	DAY 22	DAY 23	DAY 24	DAY 25	DAY 26	DAY 27	DAY 28	DAY 29	DAY 30

MEAL PLAN

DAY 1	DAY 2	DAY 3	DAY 4	DAY 5	DAY 6	DAY 7	DAY 8	DAY 9	DAY 10
DAY 11	DAY 12	DAY 13	DAY 14	DAY 15	DAY 16	DAY 17	DAY 18	DAY 19	DAY 20
DAY 21	DAY 22	DAY 23	DAY 24	DAY 25	DAY 26	DAY 27	DAY 28	DAY 29	DAY 30

30 Day Wellness Tracker

MONTH: _____

SLEEP

DAY 1	DAY 2	DAY 3	DAY 4	DAY 5	DAY 6	DAY 7	DAY 8	DAY 9	DAY 10
DAY 11	DAY 12	DAY 13	DAY 14	DAY 15	DAY 16	DAY 17	DAY 18	DAY 19	DAY 20
DAY 21	DAY 22	DAY 23	DAY 24	DAY 25	DAY 26	DAY 27	DAY 28	DAY 29	DAY 30

SELF CARE ROUTINE

DAY 1	DAY 2	DAY 3	DAY 4	DAY 5	DAY 6	DAY 7	DAY 8	DAY 9	DAY 10
DAY 11	DAY 12	DAY 13	DAY 14	DAY 15	DAY 16	DAY 17	DAY 18	DAY 19	DAY 20
DAY 21	DAY 22	DAY 23	DAY 24	DAY 25	DAY 26	DAY 27	DAY 28	DAY 29	DAY 30

EXERCISE

DAY 1	DAY 2	DAY 3	DAY 4	DAY 5	DAY 6	DAY 7	DAY 8	DAY 9	DAY 10
DAY 11	DAY 12	DAY 13	DAY 14	DAY 15	DAY 16	DAY 17	DAY 18	DAY 19	DAY 20
DAY 21	DAY 22	DAY 23	DAY 24	DAY 25	DAY 26	DAY 27	DAY 28	DAY 29	DAY 30

MEAL PLAN

DAY 1	DAY 2	DAY 3	DAY 4	DAY 5	DAY 6	DAY 7	DAY 8	DAY 9	DAY 10
DAY 11	DAY 12	DAY 13	DAY 14	DAY 15	DAY 16	DAY 17	DAY 18	DAY 19	DAY 20
DAY 21	DAY 22	DAY 23	DAY 24	DAY 25	DAY 26	DAY 27	DAY 28	DAY 29	DAY 30

Made in United States
Orlando, FL
05 August 2024

49966199R00134